LIVING BETTER

EVERY PATIENT'S GUIDE TO LIVING WITH ILLNESS

CAROL J. LANGENFELD, M.S., L.P.C.
AND
DOUGLAS E. LANGENFELD, M.B.A., C.P.A.

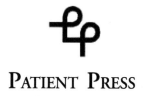

PATIENT PRESS

Published by Patient Press
6475 Perimeter Drive, Box 110
Dublin, Ohio 43016

The authors gratefully acknowledge permission to include the following copyrighted works:

Portia Nelson's poem, *There's a Hole in My Sidewalk*. Copyright © 1993 by Portia Nelson. Reprinted with permission from Portia Nelson and Beyond Words Publishing.

Selections from *Heart Illness and Intimacy* by Wayne M. Sotile, Ph.D. Copyright © 1992 by Wayne M. Sotile. Used by permission from Wayne M. Sotile.

Selections adapted from *The Healthy Mind Healthy Body Handbook* by David Sobel, M.D., and Robert Ornstein, Ph.D., published by DRx: Los Altos, California. Copyright © 1998. Available from ISHK Book Service (800/222-4745), www.ISHKBook.com. Reprinted with permission from David Sobel and DRx.

Selections from *Imagery for Getting Well* by Deirdre Davis Brigham. Copyright © 1994 by Deirdre Davis Brigham. Reprinted with her permission.

Selected materials adapted from training materials from Harvard Medical School's Mind/Body Medical Institute are included in several chapters, especially Chapter Six. Various copyright dates. Used by permission of the Mind/Body Medical Institute.

Cover photo by Carol J. Langenfeld.

Library of Congress Cataloging-in-Publication Information:
    Langenfeld, Carol J.
    Living better : every patient's guide to living with illness / Carol J. Langenfeld and Douglas E. Langenfeld.
    -- 1st ed.
        p. cm.
        Includes index.
        ISBN 0-9701545-1-8
        1. Sick--Psychology. 2. Adjustment (Psychology). 3. Mind and body. 4. Health.
        5. Self-help techniques.
        I. Langenfeld, Douglas E. II. Title.
        R726.5.L36 2001   616'.001'9
            QBI00-901164

ISBN : 0-9701545-1-8
Printed in the United States of America

Dedication

To our mothers, fathers, and stepfather, who have been our cheerleaders and supporters, helping us survive some of our toughest challenges and showing their own courage in dealing with their own and their spouses' health struggles.

To our son Eric, who has helped us see things differently because of his unique and often insightful views on life.

Table of Contents

Acknowledgments

We have many people to thank and acknowledge. We apologize in advance, for regardless of how long our list of acknowledgments, we have missed someone who has contributed significantly to the creation of this book and to our ability to live with our illnesses.

Thank you to all of our family for crying with us at each new stage of illness and for not laughing at us. We especially want to acknowledge our most immediate family, Eric Langenfeld, Bill Courtney, Mark and Kathy Langenfeld, and Ken and Cristy Jones.

We also owe a debt of thanks to Dr. Bill Salt and Susan Salt; Susan for holding our hands through the publishing process and Bill for his medical expertise, modeling the ideal physician approach to the patient-physician relationship, encouraging Carol to write a book, and writing the foreword.

We also had wonderful professional support from Robert Howard, who designed the cover, Laura Dutton, who created order out of chaos in cleaning up our word processing, and laying out the book's content, Kate Bandos, who has helped us with publicity, and Dan Poynter, who advised us on the publishing business. Lois Porter edited our book and not only cleaned up our manuscript but also helped make our message clearer and contributed some insightful content. We will not soon forget those pages full of her red-ink edit comments, in her very small handwriting.

We appreciate everyone who took time to read early drafts of our book and give us their comments and suggestions. Those reviewers include Bill and Susan Salt, Chuck Ansley, Steve Hoover, Elaine Horr, Dr. John Larrimer, Dr. Mark Langenfeld, Jim Lillibridge, Paul Miller, Dr. Jan Morrison, Lynn Pease, and Keilah Richardson. Thank you.

So many friends have touched our lives in many ways over the past twentysome years as we learned over and over again how to live with life-changing illness. These friends include "The Mariners," who know who they are but may never know just how much their hands-on ministering helped get us through times when Carol was very sick and our son was a toddler.

Our friendships with the Brinks, Polings and Harklesses go back to elementary school but have grown much deeper and closer as adults, as we shared together the challenges and struggles of our various families' illnesses and other life challenges.

Carol's share group friends Elaine, Anne, Lynn, and Debbie and her Sunday School classmates have listened to her and encouraged her through the process of writing and publishing this book and with our life struggles.

Our friend Jean Goldsmith's warm and caring words and actions have been our "chicken soup" since long before the famous book series.

Many, many ministers and church members at Brookwood Presbyterian, Holy Redeemer Lutheran and Indian Run United Methodist Churches have helped us through good times and hard times. They helped us learn and relearn how to reconcile the frustrations of life's challenges with our continuing strong faith in an infinitely loving God.

Foreword

I am certain that most people take health for granted, and that very few view health as an active rather than a passive process—at least until they are faced with a life-threatening chronic disease and illness. Circumstances that are usually beyond their control impose a new life direction that includes pain, symptoms, and emotional distress ranging from high anxiety to low despair and depression. The future becomes much more uncertain than ever before. Suddenly, people become patients and enter the strange, uncomfortable and frankly risky world of doctors and hospitals. Control seems lost; yet, multiple decisions must be made in the face of constant uncertainty.

Carol and Doug Langenfeld know all of this, because they live it. I have had the great privilege to know Carol and Doug for more than 20 years now as one of their physicians and as a friend. Each has a serious chronic disease that threatens life and is unlikely to be biomedically cured. Carol has scleroderma and has had several near death experiences. As her health gained some stability, Carol completed graduate school and became a highly skilled mental health counselor. Recently she has chosen to scale back her busy counseling practice and redirect her life because she could not meet the physical demands required without jeopardizing her health or compromising her patients' health because of her own limitations. Doug is a talented C.P.A. specializing in health care who was forced to retire from partnership in an international accounting and consulting firm because of a pituitary tumor that has caused acromegaly, heart arrhythmia, headaches, and visual problems.

Chronic disease and illness have changed the lives of Carol and Doug and led them to a true appreciation and understanding of Mind-Body-Spirit healing. They understand the miracle of free will to choose their attitudes, thoughts, beliefs, and behaviors. They accept their responsibility to be in charge of their own health.

The eminent psychiatrist, Viktor Frankl, was imprisoned at Auschwitz and other concentration camps for three years during the Second World War. He began to study why some of his fellow prisoners were not only able to survive the horrifying conditions, but also to grow in the process. In the book, *Man's Search for Meaning*, he concluded that, "Man is not destroyed by suffering. He is destroyed by suffering without meaning."

Carol and Doug know that chronic disease and illness provide the opportunity to choose exploration of life's meaning in order to relieve suffering. They know that healing is an ongoing and active pursuit that does not necessarily include biomedical cure of disease. They choose to share their experience and advice in this marvelous book for all who suffer with chronic disease and illness and aspire to find meaning and healing.

William B. Salt II, M.D.
Author of *Irritable Bowel Syndrome & the Mind-Body/Brain-Gut Connection*
Co-author of *Fibromyalgia and the MindBodySpirit Connection*
(Both published by Parkview Publishing)

FACING YOUR ILLNESS AND MAKING NEW CHOICES

Two roads diverged in a wood, and I,
I took the one less traveled by,
And that has made all the difference.

– Robert Frost

We came face-to-face with illness in 1979. We may have been too young to know it then, but we were at the point where two roads diverged. One road would have led us to unhealthy choices such as denying that Carol's disease was real. Instead, we made a choice to take the road that led us to find opportunities hidden within the crisis Carol's illness presented. We found friends, family, and faith that we might not have otherwise discovered. We found inner strength and capabilities we never could have imagined. That road eventually led us to write this book.

We have written this book from a patient's perspective, as patients to patients. We started our trip down the curvy, bumpy road of chronic illness more than 20 years ago. If you or someone very close to you are in

1

the very early stages of dealing with an illness, you would be amazed how well you will remember those moments several years from now. We remember them well.

Although our illness can be accurately called chronic illness, we prefer a more descriptive and positive adjective: *life-changing*. Here is our definition of life-changing illness:

> Life-changing illness is an illness that is the result of diseases and/or conditions that have a dramatic, often long-term impact on how you live your life. Such an illness may or may not be life-threatening. Life-changing illness ebbs and flows, posing new challenges and bringing out new emotions. Problems come and go, but they seldom get resolved easily or fully.

If that definition fits your situation, this book is for you. This introduction tells you about our philosophy, briefly tells you "our stories," and explains why this book may be beneficial for you.

Our Philosophy

We strongly believe in the power of knowledge and self-care. Patients must play a key role in helping to shape and direct their medical treatment. It is easy to become passive and to be "taken care of" when one is sick. However, from our experience we recognize the benefits of being informed, active participants in our health care. These benefits include better medical care, a greater feeling of empowerment, and an improved lifestyle.

We also firmly believe in the mysterious and powerful links between the mind, body, and spirit in the healing process. We wrote this book at the urging of Dr. William B. Salt II, our gastroenterologist, author, and friend, who shares a similar philosophy regarding the role of the patient and the mind-body-spirit connection. We have seen him demonstrate this philosophy for more than 20 years in the way he asks questions, listens, and encourages patients.

We believe we have the credentials to write this book for you. Carol is a counselor by training and profession. Her writing is strongly influenced both by her counseling and by her experience as a survivor of a life-changing illness. Doug is a self-employed writer and investment planner who was diagnosed with a pituitary tumor in 1991, which required surgery and radiation treatments and which has resulted in continuing endocrine system complications.

Although we don't know you or your situation personally, we believe that our life experiences have given us a pretty good understanding of the road that you might be traveling. We wouldn't pretend to know how you feel, but if you are picking up this book, we assume that you or somebody close to you is struggling with an illness that you would like to manage or learn skills to cope with it.

Carol's Story

People tell me that I have earned my credentials the hard way for more than 20 years. Many times I have wished I could drop my diseased body off at the laundry and pick it up the next day, fresh and clean and ready to face the world anew.

The birth of our son, Eric, was a joyful occasion, an experience to celebrate and feel grateful. But, six weeks after his birth I could hardly pick him up. My hands were painful, hot, and swollen so that I could not shut them. I frequently opened and closed my hands to try to relax the stiffness, hoping that the pain would ease so that I could safely pick him up, unpin his diaper, change him and feed him.

Diagnosis was not easy. The test results did not fit into a diagnosis—I looked fine on paper! Eventually, my family doctor called my condition rheumatoid arthritis. But I knew that didn't really fit my symptoms. His treatments were not very helpful and I continued to get worse. Friends and family urged me to go to a specialist. I resisted but eventually, a year later, agreed to see a rheumatologist. This doctor looked at me and immediately recognized that I had a connective tissue disease called scleroderma. If you've never heard of this disease, you are not alone. I had never heard of scleroderma. Very few people are aware of this disease. Very few people have been diagnosed as having the disease. The Scleroderma Foundation estimates that 300,000 persons in the United States have scleroderma (www.scleroderma.org). I often tell friends that scleroderma is a "cousin of lupus" because people are much more likely to have heard of lupus.

This life-changing illness hit me in the first several years of my son's life. I was young, in my early and middle 20s. Though doctors and researchers may have more specific explanations and understandings about this disease, what I knew at the time was that I desperately hurt. I was always cold. My hands were blue. I had terrible "acid indigestion." Swallowing was painful. Breathing deeply made my chest ache.

In addition, I began to frequently feel strange palpitations in my chest. Eventually, I blacked out at home and my family called the emergency squad to take me to the emergency room. Six weeks later, after confirming that my heart did not reliably conduct the electrical impulse to cause my heart to beat, I had surgery to implant a cardiac pacemaker. That was the beginning of some life-threatening events that still happen occasionally.

Today, I still have scleroderma (although it is in remission) and its residual damage. And now more than 20 years later I still occasionally have aches and pains. I take eight to ten different prescriptions – give or take a few depending on the day – and I still take a nap on most days. In addition, I am still totally dependent on the cardiac pacemaker to keep my heart from stopping.

With the help and encouragement of many, many friends and family, I have nonetheless been a mother for 23 years and a wife for 25 years. I completed my Master's degree in social agency counseling in 1996 and now work part-time.

Doug's Story

I have lived through Carol's delicate medical condition for more than 20 years. Generally, this has meant living day in and day out with a chronic, life-changing illness. On several occasions, Carol's health has erupted in crisis—truly life-threatening situations.

More recently, my story has moved me from a supporting role into a lead character, "the patient." In May, 1991, I saw our family physician, Dr. Joseph Carducci, and complained about the constant headaches that I had tried to ignore for at least a year. He listened to me describe my symptoms. He asked me many questions and he noted my yellowish skin color and sharpened facial features. I later learned that he strongly suspected a pituitary tumor.

He ordered tests—including a computerized tomography (CT or CAT) scan, magnetic resonance imaging (MRI) and others. The results confirmed Dr. Carducci's suspicions and helped pinpoint the location of the tumor, which gave the surgeon a detailed road map for surgery. The

11-day wait to see Dr. Sadar, the neurosurgeon, seemed like forever. The words "probably benign" feel completely different from the single word "benign." Once I saw Dr. Sadar, I immediately had more tests and then surgery. While I waited, I learned that the pituitary gland is located just below the brain (very close to the optic nerve and the main arteries to the brain). I also learned that the pituitary gland tells the rest of the endocrine system when, where, and how much of key hormones to secrete.

Just a week after "successful" surgery, I was sent home from the hospital. I had an excruciating headache and severe nausea for several days. After a week at home, I returned to the hospital for two weeks with an unforgettable bad reaction to medication, which produced an "altered thought process." At times, I was pretty sure I was going crazy.

Once that complication eased, I began five weeks of daily radiation treatments to deal with the portion of the tumor that surgery could not reach. My condition also introduced me to an assortment of medications: several to replace hormones not being produced as normal, several more to suppress unintended secretions, and several others to address other complications.

I gradually returned to work, working part-time at first, gradually working up to full-time by mid-1993. I worked full-time until late 1997, when the cumulative effects of surgery, tumor, radiation, and medications, causing a lack of energy, fatigue, weakness, muscle tightness and pain, and loss of mental quickness, forced me to take disability. I gave up my position with the large company where I had worked for 23 years, recognizing that my professional career was impossible to sustain at the required break-neck pace. My family's lifestyle changed dramatically and continues to be reshaped even now.

What You Can Expect From This Book

If you or someone very close to you is dealing with a life-changing illness, this book is for you. By reading this book, you will learn how to adapt and make the most out of what is most likely a difficult situation. We will share and describe tools for your journey and include examples of how they have helped us in our journeys.

We intend for this book to be a guide for you to use in a variety of ways. You can pick it up and read it from cover to cover. You can browse through it to find some specific information you need for today.

The first four chapters deal with understanding how to navigate yourself and your illness through the healthcare world. If you have been ill for some time, you may have already mastered much of this navigational process. We may be slow learners, but we find that we are still learning and relearning how to make best use of the system to meet our medical needs. With the constantly changing healthcare environment, there always seems to be a new hurdle to jump or a new skill to master. These first four chapters focus on the world of illness outside of you.

Chapter Five focuses on taking care of your body, in light of your illness. Then, in Chapters Six through Ten, our focus shifts to learning a different way to live. You will look at your "inside" world, your lifestyle, and how you view and live your life. As a family friend said, in describing how he and his wife coped with his wife's lupus, "It requires a *different way* of living." His answer was so simple and yet so profound. We hope that this book will be a guide to help you find and define *your* different way of living.

Facing Your Illness, Making New Choices

Just by its nature, life-changing illness requires you to look inside yourself. Your life has changed. No one knows that better that you do. Your plans, as you knew them, are now on hold—at least for a while and possibly for the rest of your life. The rules by which you thought you "played" life don't exist anymore. These necessary changes do not mean you need to quit. However, they do require learning new skills and setting new goals for your life. Beginning with Chapter Five, our focus is on learning these skills and re-evaluating your goals.

You are a very complex and unique system. As one part of you changes, your whole self will need to adapt. We believe that no matter how greatly your lifestyle is challenged by illness, you can increase your control of your life by nurturing your biological, psychological, and spiritual dimensions. We will take time to look at each of these dimensions.

Finding a different way to live is a key to understanding and tapping into the power of your mind-body connection. To say that your mind, your body, and your spirit (more in Chapter Six on the mind-body-spirit connection) are connected is really a big understatement. In truth, scientific research has begun to confirm that the mind, the body, and the spirit are not only connected but are in fact one complete process, with many components closely interacting.

Learning to use this connection can be very empowering. Patients no longer need to leave their bodies at the complete mercy of doctors, hospitals, and tests. You can begin to do your own self-care, which is just what it sounds like—taking an active role in shaping your health care and your life.

Your illness is life-changing; learning new self-care skills and reconnecting your mind, body, and spirit can play vital roles in improving your health and your overall quality of life. Why not be an active player in shaping the changes in your life by making new choices for your new situation of now living with your illness?

We wish we knew each of you and your stories. If we did, we could modify what we say to fit your specific needs. Nonetheless, you can take what we have to offer, squeeze it, stretch it, and mold it to find just how our ideas on personal wellness from our perspective as patients will fit you best. We wish you the very best as you take your own journey toward wholeness, equipped with these suggestions that we have been practicing, or at least trying to practice, for more than 20 years.

ONE

DEFINING YOUR SITUATION

Illness is an event that makes a painful difference

in the world we take for granted.

– Robert Shuman

Most people take health for granted. People who live with illness take nothing for granted. When illness enters your life, it is not only an unexpected visitor, but also a force that changes the world you live in. You may feel like you are traveling in a foreign land. And as Robert Shuman suggests, your illness makes a painful difference.

We will cover the following topics in this chapter:

- Change Happens

- Medical Miracles

- You Are Still You

- What Is Illness? How Are Illness and Disease Different?

- What is Stress and Why Is Illness So Stressful?

- Emotional Overload

- Normal Reactions to Emotional Overload

- Can Your Life Be Reconstituted?

- What Does Your Future Look Like?

Illness comes in many forms, shapes, and sizes. We know that your illness may have changed your life dramatically. For some of you, this change has happened suddenly. For others, the change has happened gradually over days, months, or years.

As a traveler in the land of life-changing illness, there are some fairly universal realities of life to consider. You are in new, unknown, and uncharted territory. Dramatic change has taken place in your life. You feel strong emotions, most of which are probably normal. People around you will tend to either overreact or underreact to your changes. You face many new challenges. These statements probably ring true for you. They may even seem like understatements of your particular situation.

Fortunately, there are some offsetting truths, some good news. First, you can take at least some control of your situation. You can make choices about your healthcare treatment and how you live your life. You can learn new skills to help yourself. You—yes, you—still have a large influence on the fullness of your life. You can be "reconstituted". Finally, you do not need to travel the road alone.

Change Happens

When illness comes, it tends to bring unexpected, sudden turns in your life. Medical science and popular culture have heightened expectations of wonderful biological remedies to "fix us up as good as new." But the problem is reality—the reality

> *The web of our life is a mingled yarn, good and ill together.*
>
> – Shakespeare

that often you are not as good as new. Your life as you knew it may have changed forever because of your life-changing illness.

When Carol was first diagnosed with scleroderma at age 25, most of our friends expected that she would have an operation or be given a pill that would "cure" the scleroderma, much like the way we take penicillin to kill strep throat bacteria. It was hard for friends and for us to understand and accept that there wasn't a cure-all fix.

Carol realized several years later that the medical community did not always have an answer. Knowing that, she began to accept more fully that her lifestyle and plans, and her family's lifestyle and plans, were going to change dramatically—forever! We weren't going to have more children; our family size was going to stay at three. Carol's physical limitations would determine the size and style of house we live in. These limitations would also influence vacations and many other aspects of our life. Our first question for many years was, "Will Carol be able do it?" You and your family may have had similar thoughts.

If cancer strikes you, you will probably never look at life the same again either. For many cancer victims, beliefs about life are shaken to the core. Paradoxically, chemotherapy heals while at the same time, it tears one's body, mind, and spirit apart. A cancer survivor always wonders if the next checkup at the doctor's will be "okay."

Heart problems often start with a heart attack. If you are a heart patient, you and your loved ones endure the immediate crisis and fear that begins in the Emergency Room and Cardiac Care Unit (CCU). Suddenly you are lying on a very uncomfortable table exposed to many strangers, wondering and asking questions, like "Am I going to die?," "How will I be remembered?", and "Is what I am presently doing worthwhile?" Then, with some medical "mumbo jumbo," doctors clean out your arteries, roto-rooter style, put in new arteries in open-heart surgery, or install battery-powered cardiac pacemakers.

Does the medical intervention cause you to stop asking the questions in the last paragraph? Probably not. These questions tend to linger as you pick up the pieces of your changed life.

Medical Miracles

We live in an age when new medical miracles, such as organ transplants and bionic devices implanted inside the body, seem to be announced almost every day. Often, however, after medicine repairs you, you are released from the hospital with a send-off, something like this: "You look like you are in good shape now, go on and live your life." Unfortunately, few doctors and other medical professionals talk to you about the emotional and physical adaptations and changes you need to make. They often fail to discuss these issues with you because of time constraints or lack of experience in discussing these issues.

Medical miracles, such as cancer therapies and heart surgery, often leave scars in places where you don't want them. For example, open-heart surgery may be deemed medically successful, but every time you get out of the shower and look in the mirror, forever, you can't escape seeing scars on your chest. Medical miracles may also bring with them emotional scars that no one but you will ever see. You may both feel and look very different.

Medical miracles may give you your life back, but not without major life changes and adjustments for you and your family. Often there is too little acknowledgment of the adjustments that you must make within yourself and the world around you. For example, if your illness prevents you from having the children you had planned, that is a major adjustment that is visible only to you and those people who know you best.

You Are Still You

After receiving a modern medical miracle, in the hospital or doctor's office, you go home. But even after you go home, you cannot escape the reality—you are still a citizen of the "kingdom of the sick," a new unknown and uncharted territory, as described by Susan Sontag in *Illness as Metaphor and AIDS and Its Metaphors*: "Everyone who is born holds dual citizenship, in the kingdom of the well and in the kingdom of the sick. Although we all prefer to use only the good passport, sooner or later each of us is obliged, at least for a spell, to identify ourselves as citizens of that other place." (Anchor Reprint, 1990.)

Most often, despite the encouraging send-off, your life will never be the same. Your lifestyle will need to change and your outlook on the world will likely need to change, too.

All is not gloom, though. Christopher Reeve's book, *Still Me* (New York: Ballantine Books, 1999), is aptly named. His wife Dana told him shortly after his tragic accident and paralysis, "You are still you." Like Reeve, even though your life is undergoing major changes, you are still you. It is helpful to learn to know who you are, what you need, and what your wishes are. You may need to endure and adapt emotionally and physically for the rest of your life. You still have the power to be positive and to take charge of your life and your medical care as much as possible.

To a greater or lesser extent, you are likely to see life through a new lens. The color of your lens to the world can help determine whether you view only danger or both danger and opportunity in your life. In Chapter Nine, "Realigning Your Attitude," we will discuss different ways you can choose to view your new world. Your attitude and the ways that you equip yourself to deal with a sudden change in your road will make a tremendous difference in the quality of your journey.

What Is Illness? How Are Illness and Disease Different?

People often confuse illness with disease. Many scientific words can be used to describe your disease. Laboratory measurements confirm a certain disease. How your body feels and what you are able to do or not do is your illness, regardless of the scientific words about your disease. You can often have a significant impact on how much your life is changed and how your lifestyle is affected by your body's disease. By learning to know yourself and care for yourself, you will learn new ways to adapt.

> *Illness is the experience of living through the disease.*
>
> – Arthur Frank

Dr. William B. Salt II describes the difference between an illness and a disease as follows: "A disease is an identifiable abnormality of the body. An illness is a person's perception of ill health. There can be a remarkable discordance between disease and illness, because they are not the same." (*Irritable Bowel Syndrome & the Mind-Body Brain-Gut Connection*, Columbus: Parkview Publishing, 1997, p. 11.)

Dr. Salt uses irritable bowel syndrome (IBS) to illustrate the difference between illness and disease. IBS has no visible abnormalities that can be described on a laboratory report. By the definition above, it is not a disease. But people with IBS know or suspect that something is very wrong with their bodies because they do not perform in the normally expected manner. Therefore, IBS is most certainly an illness.

Similarly, fibromyalgia is difficult to see in laboratory tests but can affect a sufferer in many ways. Fibromyalgia and IBS are definitely life-changing for many people, even though not life-threatening. IBS can affect what foods you are able to eat and when you feel comfortable going to social outings.

Before you receive test results, you, your friends, and your family may fear the worst, including life-threatening diseases such as an untreatable cancer. When the medical tests come back "normal," friends and family may think that the person with IBS or fibromyalgia is "just complaining" and that nothing is wrong. Nothing is further from the truth; like it or not, your lifestyle must still change to accommodate your illness. Even though Carol's scleroderma initially presented no abnormal test results, she clearly had an illness, which required treatment.

We have written this book primarily from a perspective of illness rather than disease. Reinhold Neibuhr's *Serenity Prayer* (to the right) contains great insight. Regardless of your prognosis for the future or what

> *God grant me the serenity to accept the things I cannot change, courage to change the things that I can, and wisdom to know the difference.*

your physician says has or hasn't shown up on test results, how you feel and what you think constitute your illness. You can cope with your illness every day by altering your lifestyle and improving your self-care. Change and acceptance can produce a new life opportunity within the new structure that your illness provides for you.

Every patient's situation falls somewhere on the illness/disease continuum, depending on its life-threatening nature. We have already discussed IBS, which is at one end of the continuum, not at all life-threatening. AIDS and terminal cancer are at the other end—the end of one's life is in clear sight. In between are many other illnesses, including back pain, headaches, diabetes, arthritis, other connective tissue diseases, multiple sclerosis, heart diseases, lung diseases, mental illness and many others. No matter what name your illness has, it can seriously change your life and lifestyle.

What Is Stress? Why Is Illness So Stressful?

What makes the changes brought on by illness so stressful? Dr. Margaret Caudill describes stress as "the perception of a physical or psychological threat and the perception of being ill-prepared to cope with the threat." (Margaret Caudill, M.D., Ph.D., *Managing Pain Before It Manages You,* Boston: The Guilford Press, 1995, pp. 38-39.) Note the key word: *perception.* When you view yourself as having inadequate coping skills, you are very likely to feel stressed. Most people were not taught coping skills for dealing with life-changing illness. Therefore, it is natural to perceive your life with disease as threatening and thus stressful.

Stress happens every day of your life and comes from many sources. Whether you are healthy or sick, your family, friends, and co-workers all place expectations on you. When you perceive that you cannot meet their expectations, you feel "stress." It does not matter whether your perceptions are accurate or not. The expression "reality is perception" certainly applies here. Needless to say, with life-changing illness you often cannot begin to meet expectations you previously were able to meet.

Good stress and bad stress produce the same physical response within your body. Our bodies were hard-wired to respond with a fight-or-flight response to situations we perceive to be beyond our ability to cope. Back in the era of cavemen and saber-tooth tigers, the fight-or-flight response was necessary. Today, this bodily response is often not particularly helpful. These physical responses can actually make your body sick or more susceptible to illness. We will say more about this reaction in Chapter Six, "Understanding Your Mind-Body Connection."

You may have very valid perceptions of impending threat to your lifestyle, your income, your ability to maintain control, and your independence. These are some of the reasons that illness may be so stressful for you and your loved ones. These changes often will force you to adapt. The adaptations you must make are often innumerable and ongoing— sometimes sudden and unexpected. Seldom is anyone adequately prepared by life to cope on an ongoing basis with the major changes created by a life-changing illness.

Now may be the time to take your first positive step forward, but you may not know where to start in adapting to the changes taking place in your life. Being aware of potential threats, while also seeing yourself as being unable or ill-prepared to cope with them, is indeed very stressful. When your life gets overwhelmed with many stressful events, you may feel like your life is out of control. By discovering and identifying your needs and taking positive steps, even small steps, you can help avoid the feeling of being overwhelmed. And, you can take control!

Doug describes one of his experiences with stress.

Shortly after arriving at Eric's baseball game at June 1991, I found out that something more than a headache was wrong with me. Carol said, "I have a message for you from your doctor. He wants you to see a neurosurgeon. A mass of some kind showed up on your CAT scan. He said it is most probably not cancer and not to worry."

I was shocked and numb. I didn't know what to think. Carol was in denial of the impending changes in our lives that this could mean and buried her emotions, almost pretending that nothing was wrong. She feared that doing otherwise would have allowed uncontrollable fear to take over, which she believed she could not let happen.

I had questions, but nobody to ask. While we waited the 11 days that seemed like forever to see the surgeon recommended by our family physician, I didn't know what was wrong. I just knew that a CAT scan showed a mass inside my head and that my doctor thought it was probably a 'benign' tumor on the pituitary gland. I didn't know whether or not I had cancer. I didn't know how long I would be off work and when I would be able to return to work. Without the Internet as we know it today, I couldn't easily find out much about pituitary tumors. To be honest, I wasn't sure I wanted to know much more.

Here is a sample of what I was thinking and how I was feeling, from my journal a few days before my surgery.

> *There's something unexplained inside my head.*
> *I think that's what the doctor said.*
> *I don't have any answers, just questions.*
> *How should I feel? Who should I tell?*
> *But what do I know, so what could I say?*
> *Did they misread the scan? What might it be? Should I be scared?*
> *I don't have answers, just questions.*

Feeling in control is a powerful antidote to stress. Mind-body medicine pioneer Dr. Herbert Benson sees medical care as a three-legged stool. The three legs in his model are (1) pharmaceuticals, (2) medical procedures, including surgery, and (3) self-care.

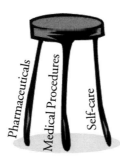

Self-care is the part of Benson's three-legged model where patients have the most control. By realizing that you have this control and learning how to make the best use of self-care, you can improve your life. Improvement often does not mean good physical health. Instead, it means improvement of your quality of life through lifestyle changes.

Emotional Overload

As you probably have discovered already, the challenges of life-changing illness are often compounded by other factors. These factors may include isolation due to the inability to drive a car or to be around people due to your fear of contracting a disease. Illness can bring changes that alter your hopes and dreams. Fear of losing your job can also contribute to your perception of helplessness and change how you identify yourself.

The onset of your illness can trigger intense emotional reactions. You may feel overwhelmed and your thoughts may be disorganized. Feeling threatened or numb is natural and normal. Feeling angry can also be normal. Sometimes Carol gets angry over something that makes no sense to an observer, but deep down the anger is coming out as a response to her illness, not the observed event. You may feel that you are not well prepared to cope with the changes; your coping skills from the past may not work now.

These changes can make you feel totally out of control. The fact that many illnesses don't have a definable end, the lack of energy caused by the disease, and the stress from the accompanying illness can create much strain on you and your family. These factors may contribute to emotional overload. Chapters Six through Ten cover new skills to cope with the emotional overload caused by your illness.

You may feel like you are going through a crisis. You are! One of the definitions of crisis is "turning point." Your chronic illness may represent a significant turning point in your life. Emotional overload is not unexpected; it is a normal response to an abnormally stressful situation. Using your illness and the danger it presents in a way that turns it into an opportunity may sound like a conflict. When Carol was first sick, no one could have told her that scleroderma was an opportunity. Looking back with 20/20 hindsight, opportunities did come. This book is an obvious example.

Normal Reactions to Emotional Overload

Emotional overload is a common response to illness, especially at its onset or during flare-ups. When you reach emotional overload, you may feel unable and inadequate to do your job as a parent, employee, or friend. You may feel even worse that you feel inadequate! Normal reactions to the losses created by your illness may include shock, denial, anger, sadness, fear, bargaining, and eventually acceptance and resolution.

These reactions are similar to the stages of grieving a death. In many ways, you have experienced death—the death of life as you knew it. These reactions do not necessarily progress in a nice, predictable, or logical order. Sometimes, just when you think that you have accepted changes in your life journey, anger or sadness will blindside you. When your reaction to an event does not fit, or is out of proportion to the situation, it may be the result of unrealized emotions creeping out.

Below, Carol remembers one of those times.

I clearly remember driving to church one day to attend a program. I chose a handicap-reserved parking place at the side of the church, near the most convenient entrance. What I did not know was that the preschool used this area for unloading their students at that same time. The preschool director came running up to me and asked me to move my car, probably unaware of my handicap license plate or my health situation. I reacted angrily toward the director and was in tears. My anger and tears did not match the simple request that was made of me.

I had an opportunity later that day to tell a caring, listening friend about the incident and my anger. What I realized was that I was angry, but not about the preschool director's request. I was angry about my husband's recently diagnosed illness. More importantly, I discovered that my fears about a situation that was totally out of my control were just below the surface, underneath my anger.

I was also surprised when I surfaced other emotions beneath my anger. I was hurt that I couldn't just be like everyone else. I was sad that my son had to worry now about his father's health in addition to mine. I had fear because not only was I dealing with my own illness, but now my husband had his own illness to deal with. What most of my friends and support people did not know was that I relied on my husband for much of what my son and I needed. Much of my lifestyle depended on him to help with things I could not do myself. Until then, he had expended energy where I could not. He had "picked up the slack." He was able to maintain a job when I could not. He had kept our life fairly "normal" for our son. Now, even *that* "normal" life appeared to be gone.

That day, anger, hurt, fear, sadness, and other emotions broke through the surface of my smiling face of denial. That day I became painfully aware of those emotions, triggered by a totally unrelated event.

When you are ill, you experience loss of important aspects of your lifestyle. Particularly painful losses can include diet changes, dramatic shifts in responsibilities, accepting physical changes and challenges, needing to change jobs or careers, or even giving up a career altogether. Understanding the grief process as we mentioned earlier is helpful. Being able to identify those feelings is necessary so that you can harness them and use them to your advantage. When Carol was aware of her fears, she could begin to problem solve and reevaluate the importance of demands in her life. She could begin to adapt to the new realities of her life, including the need to change the way she managed her housekeeping and child-care responsibilities.

Most likely, none of this is new information to you. We hope you find affirmation of the normalcy of many of the thoughts and feelings you may have experienced. Sometimes, stress triggered by your illness can make you wonder if you are going crazy. It can be very helpful to have someone tell you that you are not crazy. Although illness can make you feel like you are losing your mind, let us assure you that you are not. And you are not crazy now! In fact, as described by one of Carol's professors, Dr. Tom Rueth of the University of Dayton, you are being "reconstituted."

Can Your Life Be Reconstituted?

Absolutely! What does it mean to be reconstituted? Well, think of orange juice. Natural, freshly squeezed orange juice is absolutely wonderful. But you can also buy a can of frozen, concentrated orange juice, follow the directions to add water, and still have a very good beverage. The frozen variety may not be quite the same as freshly squeezed orange juice, but it is still very good. Just as orange juice can be reconstituted, so can you! Your life can still be "good."

There are many ways you can reconstitute your life. You can put on a new pair of glasses to look at life with a new focus. You can learn how to communicate better with your doctor. You can learn the skills you need to help you navigate through the medical system. You can learn healthy lifestyle choices. You can reach out to someone else who needs help with a new perspective on what it feels like to need that help. After accepting the dangers your illness presents, you can recognize the opportunities as well.

> *When written in Chinese, the word crisis is composed of two characters. One represents danger and the other represents opportunity.*
>
> – John F. Kennedy

Redefining what has meaning in your life and gaining knowledge about where you want to go are very important. How can you get to a better place if you don't even know where it is or what it looks like? By finding new supports and learning how to enlist them, you can redefine your life into a lifestyle with which you can cope. Skills for understanding yourself and for managing the stress are important skills to keep in your hip pocket.

Two things are certain about life-changing illness: (1) the importance of endurance and (2) the certainty of unpredictability. But the closer you keep yourself in touch with your coping skills, the more readily you will be able to access them and help avoid or minimize stress when new changes occur. This book offers some specific, concrete ideas and approaches to do this.

What Does Your Future Look Like?

Every patient's illness is unique, as are your quality of life, your support systems, and many other factors. However, there are a few common

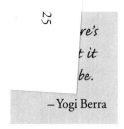

re's
t it
be.

— Yogi Berra

truths we mentioned, at the beginning of this chapter that we believe apply to most, if not all, patients with life-changing illness. You are in new, unknown, and uncharted territory, probably feel strong emotions, and face many new challenges.

Fortunately, as we mentioned there is also good news.

- You can take control.

- You can make choices and learn new skills.

- You have a large influence on the fullness of your life.

- You can be "reconstituted."

- Most importantly, you do not need to travel the road alone.

As we said earlier in defining it, life-changing illness tends to ebb and flow, bringing up new challenges and bringing to light new emotions. Problems come and go, but they seldom get resolved easily. Carol often feels like she has found resolution only to have some new problem hit her over the head and take her understanding of her life back to "square one."

We experienced going back to "square one" early in 1999 when Carol was hospitalized five times for cardiac rhythm and other heart complications of her scleroderma. Throughout these hospitalizations our endurance and resiliency were tested again. In some ways, our prior experience helped us through the crises in 1999. In other ways 1999 was more difficult because it caused us to "replay the tapes" from some of our early medical crises more than 20 years ago, bringing back old emotions of fear and anger. Some of our coping resources were gone. Family members who had so visibly supported us in earlier crises were no longer living. Others had moved far away. Fortunately, nobody needs to be alone when faced with a life-changing illness. You, your family and friends, support groups, your doctors, other resources in the medical community are also part of your team.

As you read this book, let us be a part of your team. Take each suggestion with you that will help you on your journey. The phrase "life is a journey, not a destination" applies to illness. Living with your illness is a journey, not a destination. The chapters that follow are intended to give you an idea where you are going and what to pack for the journey.

You have to take it as it happens, but you should try
to make it happen the way you want to take it.

– Old German Proverb

TWO

Developing a Partnership with Your Healthcare Team

A doctor who cannot take a good history and a patient who cannot give one are in danger of giving and receiving bad advice.

– Paul Dudley White. M.D.

*D*eveloping a truly collaborative partnership with your doctor and other healthcare professionals makes a huge difference in how effectively your medical team addresses your medical issues. Most doctors are dedicated, highly skilled, and caring professionals. Yet many people feel intimidated by doctors. We do not deny that some doctors and other healthcare professionals, and perhaps the entire medical complex, can be very intimidating. Even the doctors' white coats can evoke strong emotions, including raising some people's blood pressure. Nonetheless, overcoming intimidation and fear is essential to your being able to communicate effectively with your doctor.

This chapter provides practical tips for building a good working relationship with your doctor. Topics include the following:

- What Is a Patient?

- Your Rights as a Patient

- Who Is in Charge?

- How Can You Change Your Mind-Set?

- Knowledge Is Power

- What Knowledge Do You Need?

- How Do You Acquire the Knowledge You Need?

- Making the Best Use of Limited Time with Your Doctor

- Good Patient, Bad Patient

- When Do You Need a Second Opinion?

- Summary

What Is a Patient?

A good place to start in developing a relationship with anyone in the medical world is to define the word *patient*. Lying in a hospital bed with too much time to think, Doug once noticed the surprising similarity of two words: *patient* (noun) and *patient* (adjective). (You may have already noticed that they are spelled exactly the same.) What does it mean to be a patient? Consider the following dictionary definitions:

pa tient (pa' shent) noun. 1: a person who is being treated by a doctor. 2: a person or thing that undergoes some action; recipient.

pa tient (pa' shent) adjective. 1: willing to put up with waiting, pain, or anything that annoys, troubles, or hurts; enduring calmly without complaining or losing self-control.

(*The World Book Dictionary*, Chicago: World Book, Inc., 2000, p. 1527.)

While the definition of the noun is accurate, note the lack of any active role. The second definition, as an adjective, conveys a strong message about the importance of calmly putting up with uncomfortable events and surroundings. But note again the lack of an active role.

We believe that both of these definitions are missing a key component of being a patient—the patient as an active partner on the medical treatment team. We suggest you consider this proposed definition as you think about what kind of patient you want to be:

pa tient (pa' shent) noun. 1: a well-informed person who seeks knowledge, forms an effective partnership with doctors and other healthcare professionals and makes decisions that help to shape his or her treatment.

As a patient, you can gain knowledge about your disease and your treatment options. You can also get to know your doctors and other members of your medical team. You can balance the reality of your disease with preventing the disease from defining you. You can recognize that you are a customer. Although you are probably not a medical expert, you are equipped with the knowledge and power to make choices. You do not need to be a passive, inactive recipient of treatment.

You can be patient, too. Patience is a wonderful alternative to anxiety! But clearly, being an effective patient requires much more than just being patient.

Your Rights as a Patient

As our new definition of *patient* implies, you do have rights. We will cover patient rights more fully in the next chapter. For the time being, keep in mind that you do have some important rights.

You have the right to understand the pros and cons of any medical treatment before you agree to it. You also have the right to say "no" to a proposed treatment and request an alternative. Your medical records are yours. Though access may not always be easy, you have the right to see your records, including x-rays and lab reports.

In addition, you have the right to be treated considerately and respectfully. While being a patient often requires you to compromise your privacy, you still have the right to be treated with dignity. You have the right to hospital services if you need them, regardless of your ability to pay. This right is supported by federal laws governing the Medicare and Medicaid programs.

Finally, you have the right to direct that you not be resuscitated or have extreme measures taken to extend your life. See also the section "Know Your Rights and Responsibilities" in Chapter Three.

Who Is in Charge?

In one word, YOU. You are in charge. We do not mean in any way to imply that you should not place high value on your doctor's knowledge.

There is no way you can or should try to out-doctor your doctor. However, it is important not to forget who is paying the bill or paying the health insurance premiums that the insurance company uses to pay medical claims. Yet even people who otherwise tend to take charge forget that they are the customer when they visit the doctor.

Recognizing that you are the customer is important. If you are struggling with that concept, we encourage you to rethink your view of the doctor-patient relationship so that you begin to view yourself as at least an equal partner in your care. We think you will find that view to be empowering.

How Can You Change Your Mind-Set?

If you are having trouble with the concept of being more of an equal with your doctor, try the following illustration to help you make this change in attitude.

Imagine that you are the owner of very expensive racing car. You happen to be a professional driver as well. You have a greater investment in the vehicle, its performance, and its safety than anyone else. You have the most at stake if something goes wrong with the car. You feel the implications much more than anyone else. Now imagine that the expensive racing car is your body. You are the owner. You are the driver. You have the most at stake. You call the shots.

Next, you hire a crew chief, a highly skilled professional who knows how to fine-tune the vehicle to get around the track quickly and safely. You use your crew chief's intelligence, knowledge, and physical abilities to fine-tune your vehicle. The crew chief is your doctor, at least when you are at the track—the physician's office or other medical facility.

An owner, a car, a driver, and a crew chief still need a crew. Each member must have a clearly defined role and work together as a team to keep the car in the race. This highly synchronized team, which is most visible during pit stops in a race, changes tires, refuels, and makes other adjustments in a matter of seconds. The crew in this analogy is the physician's office staff, your referring doctor, and other support people. They are essential resources.

While this analogy may oversimplify roles somewhat, it serves to illustrate these key points:

- You are the owner and driver of your life, your body, and your treatment.

- You need to have a highly skilled physician who is not only very knowledgeable and competent, but also who listens to you and respects your needs as the owner/driver.

- You need to have a good crew, office and clinical support people who are competent and also listen to you and respect you as the owner.

- You all need to work as a team.

Knowledge Is Power

Much of your anxiety and possible sense of inferiority comes from the fact that doctors have a lot more medical training than most patients have. In reminding us, "You have to be your own endocrinologist," Dr. Larrimer's point is that you, the patient, know you and your illness

> *You have to be your own endocrinologist.*
>
> – John Larrimer, M.D.

better than anyone else does.

Only you know you! You know if your pain is worse than it was a month ago. You know how cold weather, hot weather, or humidity affect your pain. Only you know what aches, when it aches, and under what circumstances it aches. But there are many times when your care and treatment requires another opinion—from a real doctor.

This knowledge that *only* you have about yourself and how your body feels is very powerful. You can gain additional power by learning as much as possible about the medical side of your situation without trying to compete with your doctor.

You do not need to attempt to understand your medical situation to the same extent as your physician who has completed four years of college, three or four years of medical school, and four years or more of internships, residencies, and fellowships. However, you can learn enough to make your time spent with your physician most effective.

Knowledge gives you some power and control and it gives you the ability to make choices. If your insurance benefit permits, you have the option to make an informed decision in selecting your physicians. You have other choices, including how you want to interact with your doctor, how much you want to know, and whether and when to get a second opinion.

What Knowledge Do You Need?

Your first obstacle to overcome is that you don't know what you don't know. Dr. Timothy McCall says that if medical professionals are willing to talk about medicine in plain language, the principles about how it should be practiced are easy to understand.

We would suggest that you consider some key factors in selecting your healthcare professionals.

- **Competence.** Does he or she have the knowledge to recognize symptoms of various diseases and what tests are necessary, the skills to perform physical exams, good communications skills, and appropriate technical skills? Training and credentials give you strong indications of competency. You may be able to look at the walls in the doctor's office to see where he or she completed medical training, medical school, internships, residencies, post-residency fellowships, other special training and board certifications. Specialization is also a key factor. Knowing and understanding your doctor's area of specialization is important. You would not want an oral surgeon to work on your kneecap, for example.

  > *A good doctor treats both the patient and the illness.*
  >
  > – A Proverb

- **Philosophy of practice.** What is the doctor's attitude about involving patients in healthcare decisions? What is his or her attitude about aggressive drug therapies, surgeries, and other interventions? What is the doctor's attitude about prevention of illness and disease and about new therapies and adoption of the latest trends?

- **Bedside manner.** Does the doctor combine good listening skills with a compassionate style?

- **Taking the time to do it right.** Does the physician take the time to do a complete physical examination and to ask a lot of questions? Does he or she place a high priority on educating patients?

- **Financial considerations.** How do health plans and insurance companies compensate your doctor? You will definitely want to know and understand how the doctor is paid. Virtually all doctors keep their patients' well-being first and foremost, but you still need to understand the way a physician is paid and how that might unintentionally influence decisions regarding such key issues as referral to another specialist and which tests to order. You also want to know what incentives or disincentives the doctor receives for testing, referrals, and hospital admissions. Remember, too, that some of these decisions may have been made for you already by your health insurance plan or health maintenance organization (HMO).

- **Physical setting and environment.** What does the office look like? How does it feel? The physical setting and environment are important. Most people would prefer to see their doctor in a setting that is warm, friendly, secure, somewhat private, and equipped with fairly up-to-date technology.

- **Supporting staff.** How are you treated when you enter the office? What is the general tone and personality of the nurses and assistants? The quality and attitude of the physician's supporting staff are critical to the success of your patient-physician partnership. You need to know what level of authority and training the nurses and other medical professionals and paraprofessionals have.

- **Scheduling.** Who makes appointments? Are there multiple systems for different types of appointments and procedures? Is there something you need to know to do differently if you really, *really* need an appointment and cannot wait six or eight weeks to see the doctor? Should you have tests performed in advance of your visit to the doctor so that he or she has the results of procedures available prior to your office visit? Does the doctor generally run on time with appointments or regularly run late? Are there certain predictable times of day that are particularly good or bad for seeing the doctor on time? We have found that the first appointment of the day is probably the most likely to be on time, though still subject to emergencies.

- **Communications issues.** How are you going to be informed of test results? When does the doctor call patients? Sometimes, doctors make calls from home, at times quite late in the evening. That is worth knowing if you call in the morning and do not want to stay by the phone waiting for a call all day. Some doctors' offices are beginning to see the benefits of using e-mail as a way to reduce playing "telephone tag" with patients. As with any e-mail message, be aware that there isn't perfect privacy, so sensitive communications may not be appropriate for e-mail.

Dr. Timothy McCall describes the first four factors above—competency, philosophy, bedside manner, and taking time to do it right—as having "the largest impact on the quality of medical care." ("The Right Stuff," *Arthritis Today*, by Timothy McCall, M.D., July-August 1996, pp.17-23.)

After all is said and done, you have to find doctors and other healthcare professionals that you believe in. Dr. Herbert Benson titles one of the chapters in his book *Timeless Healing* "Trust Your Instincts, Trust Your Doctor." Dr. Benson describes how important it is to believe in your doctor, the medications, and other components of your treatment. He says, "You want someone who not only cares *for* you, but cares *about* you." (Herbert Benson, M.D., *Timeless Healing: The Power and Biology of Belief.* New York: Scribner, 1996, p. 246.) Believing in your healthcare professionals is one of the keys to the effectiveness of your care.

How Do You Acquire the Knowledge You Need?

You will need to gather knowledge from a combination of sources. Obviously, many books are available at your library or bookstore. Books, resources on the Internet, and pamphlets from your doctor's office can help in providing knowledge about your diagnosed or suspected disease.

In addition, don't forget support organizations. For example, if you have arthritis or another connective tissue disease, you can contact your local chapter of the Arthritis Foundation and request information, resources, and support for people with your disease. The same approach would apply for other diseases, including diabetes, heart disease, and cancer. You can also contact these organizations through their Web sites.

Gathering knowledge about a doctor presents more of a challenge. Probably the best advice is to ask, ask, ask. Ask friends, doctors, and other medical professionals you know. We alluded earlier to the office walls as a place where you will finds clues about the doctor's background,

> *You can observe a lot just by watching.*
>
> – Yogi Berra

training, and experience. As baseball Hall of Famer, All-Century Team catcher, and popular philosopher Yogi Berra points out (see quote), the things you observe provide an additional source of information. To find out about your doctor's board certification and similar information, you can contact services like Medi-Net (800/972-6334).

Just remember, no source of information is perfect. No doctor is perfect. Then again, neither is any patient perfect!

Making the Best Use of Limited Time with Your Doctor

Make believe that you are preparing to visit a very expensive expert whose advice you seek regarding a very expensive investment. In reality, you are! Your visit is going to be expensive. Whether you are paying for the visit directly or through insurance coverage, medical care is expensive. Your body is a very important investment. In short, you are worth the time and trouble it will require for you to be adequately prepared.

Most doctors are very busy. In fact, you would probably be uncomfortable if your doctor wasn't busy, much like you would feel in an empty restaurant at a normally busy time. Patients should generally accept the fact that doctors are busy and their time to spend with an individual patient is going to be limited. The pressures of managed care have resulted in doctors spending fewer minutes with each patient.

Your knowledge of your disease is important, as stated previously. Making the most of your time with the doctor is heavily dependent on your preparation. We recommend that you use this information to help you prepare for your visit. Try to do the following as preparation.

- **Know about your illness.** You need to learn enough about your medical condition to have a basic understanding of what is going on inside of you and how you can help yourself:

  - Learn about the most common causes.

  - Find out what drugs are available and commonly used, as well as side effects.

  - Be aware of lifestyle changes you can make that may affect the severity of your illness.

- Look into newer treatment alternatives; research what is known about their effectiveness.

- **List questions.** Put together a list of questions you want to ask the doctor. Put your questions and concerns in order of priority in case you are not able to ask all of your questions.

- **Consider questions the doctor may ask you.** Think about the questions the doctor is likely to ask. Common questions include your past medical history, when your symptoms started, your symptoms, and current medications.

Bad communications are at the heart of most of the barriers to an effective patient-health professional relationship. Patient and physician behaviors can contribute to difficulty getting to the right diagnosis. Consider the following keys to promote good use of your physician visit.

- **Communicate clearly.** Tell the doctor your principal complaint first. Speak clearly, getting to the point. Have a list of questions prepared and maybe rehearsed.

- **Make sure you understand the physician.** Repeat or paraphrase what you think the doctor said. This tactic can be very helpful in making sure you "got it." Ask for clarification. If you don't understand the answer or think the answer is inadequate, ask again or say that you don't understand.

- **Bring past records along if at all possible.** This can be a time-saver as well as improve your prospects for effective medical care.

- **Answer the doctor's questions clearly.** Too often, patients do not know how to answer a doctor's question so they respond to a different question. Stay focused. Avoid the temptation to get off track and share information that confuses the issues.

- **Don't be afraid to ask questions.** It is your right to be able to find out as much as you feel you need to know.

- **Don't allow someone to put words in your mouth.** This can happen if the patient is not providing the doctor very much information and the doctor starts to suggest symptoms. Patients will sometimes respond *yes* because they are eager to please and afraid that saying *no* is somehow the wrong answer.

- **Take notes.** If you have one, a small cassette recorder is also helpful.

- **Take along a spouse or friend.** This can be very helpful. Two sets of ears are better than one. Then after the doctor's visit you can compare notes with that person. An extra set of ears helps immeasurably in "catching" all of the important points the doctor says at a time when your brain may be on overload from the stress you are carrying with you. An added benefit, if the person you take along is a close friend or family member who tends to ask you what the doctor said, is that you don't have to answer their questions!

- **Don't hold back; volunteer information.** The doctor's office is not like a court of law! It is all right to tell the doctor something you think is important even if you are not asked the question. Also, don't consider any concern or question to be unimportant.

Finally, remember to ask about alternatives to the one being offered to you. Doctors usually do a good job presenting treatment alternatives and explaining the pros and cons of each. But it does not hurt to ask.

Asking a question, such as "What other alternatives are there?," sometimes triggers further thought by your doctor.

Good Patient, Bad Patient

Finding the right balance between being assertive and being agreeable is every patient's unique responsibility. You may get better treatment by keeping a positive outlook, joking around, and being light hearted. By human nature, people enjoy being around people who have a positive outlook more than being around complainers. Be careful, though. You do need to express your needs.

When you are a patient, being "bad" is good, if "bad" means you ask a lot of questions and expect a lot from your medical team. Dr. Bernie Siegel believes that having a "participatory relationship" with your doctor is essential and that being assertive is a key to such a relationship with your doctor. (*Love, Medicine & Miracles,* New York: Harper Row, 1986, p. 172.) By being honest and expressive, some may see you as a "bad" patient. After all, you get in the way of the regimen in hospitals and doctors' offices. But this same honesty and expression lead to getting what you need, improving your quality of care.

In *Cancer as a Turning Point,* author Lawrence LeShan contends that some medical people view a good patient as someone who accepts everything they say without question. Don't be afraid to be what LeShan calls a bad patient:

> A bad patient is one who asks questions which they do not have answers, raises problems with which they are uncomfortable, and does not accept hospital procedures as necessarily wise, useful, or intelligent. (*Cancer as a Turning Point,* New York: Penguin, 1994, p. 95.)

Amiable patients, by trying too hard to please others, do not necessarily give their doctors the best description of their condition. Being amiable is admirable, but don't keep secrets from your doctor.

When Do You Need a Second Opinion?

You need a second opinion any time you have serious doubts or reservations about the diagnosis you receive or the physician who gave you the diagnosis. However, getting a second opinion may not be as easy as it sounds. Maybe you feel uncomfortable asking for a second opinion. Even though most health insurance plans encourage you to get a second opinion, many people feel uncomfortable about raising the issue.

You Might Be Thinking...

What you say about the need for patients to take charge of their situation, assert their rights, and express their needs sounds great. But those things are really hard to do when you're sick. Sometimes, it's all I can do to get to the doctor and get home. I have often needed to ask more questions or consider getting a second opinion. But I didn't have the physical or emotional energy to do that. I was too tired to ask the extra questions or take the time and energy to go get another opinion, let alone the awkwardness of telling my doctor that I wanted to get that second opinion. So I didn't really take charge. I even ignored suggestions by family and friends. I just followed the doctor's lead.

Perhaps you know that your doctor referred you to a specialist who is a friend and long-time professional colleague of your doctor. In such a situation, you may feel awkward about making a change, even if you don't feel right about the specialist you've seen. One approach might be to tell your referring doctor, "I need to feel as secure with the specialist as I do with you." Furthermore, there are many sources of names to consider for a second opinion, including friends, neighbors, relatives, other doctors, organizations that award credentials, medical societies, and medical schools.

If there is a difference between the first and second opinions, you may need to seek a third opinion, maybe more, until you are comfortable that there is a firm consensus about your condition and about the recommended course of treatment.

...and Our Response Would Be ...

Whether it helps or not, remember that you're not alone. Many of the things you described are difficult things to do. Many patients struggle; they feel uncomfortable raising some issues. Here are several things to consider. You don't have to do any of those things if you don't want to do them. You may not want to have a second opinion. You may not want to consider a treatment approach that differs from your doctor's recommendation, and you have every right to make those choices. Nonetheless, we believe that our general advice is valid. You are most likely to get the best treatment if you can find the resources within yourself and from family or friends to take charge of your situation. Always try to remember that you know you better than anybody else does and you can use that insider knowledge to your advantage in designing the best approach to your health. Nothing in this book should be taken to imply that this is easy—because it isn't.

Summary

Finding the right doctor for you, feeling empowered and knowledgeable about your illness, and building a positive and collaborative working partnership with your doctor will go a long way toward building a successful healthcare team.

We mentioned the importance of your entire medical team working as a team in our racing car analogy, and the point is worth repeating. When your team includes doctors from different specialties and different practice groups, maybe practicing at different hospitals and in different cities, creating a seamless team effort is a difficult, but nonetheless important challenge. Ultimately, you are in charge. You may need to be a catalyst for good communication between your doctors. For example, if you are seeing more than one doctor, you might need to remind each of them who should be sent copies of letters and test results.

In Chapter Three, "Dealing with Hospitals, Tests, and Medications," we discuss many of the issues you will need to deal with as you navigate through hospitals, tests, medications, and other road hazards on your highway to wholeness.

Each patient carries his own doctor inside of him.

– Albert Schweitzer, M.D.

THREE

Dealing with Hospitals, Tests, and Medications

*Minor surgery is when they do the operation
on someone else, not you.*

— Bill Walton

No test or procedure seems minor if you are personally involved, no matter how "routine" it seems to experienced medical professionals! Such events are everyday occurrences in hospitals. We have also found that hospitals tend to be a land where a foreign language—"Medispeak"— is spoken. No matter how well you understand your native language, medical terminology can be confusing and even overwhelming.

This chapter looks at the unique experience of being a hospital patient. We have extensive experience as overnight guests (inpatients) and as day-trippers (outpatients). We have been the recipients of too many different procedures to count.

So you know where we are coming from, we don't believe that hospitals are bad places. Our philosophy is simple: when you need to be in the hospital, you need to be in the hospital. Everything else in your life and your family members' lives, must take a back seat. Quite frankly, the security of a hospital setting and proximity to medical expertise may be reassuring when your medical situation is uncertain and unstable. We also believe that everyone has the power to make the experience as pleasant and productive as possible.

We approach this chapter with the assumption that you can have a positive experience as a hospital patient and that you can develop a good understanding of the lingo and learn to tolerate the tests and procedures fairly well. Here are the topics we will cover.

- The Emergency Room Experience

- Before Going to the Hospital (Except in an Emergency)

- What to Take to the Hospital

- Check (Some of) Your Dignity at the Door

- Know Your Rights and Responsibilities

- What Should You Expect as an Inpatient?

- Visitors

- Humor Helps You Heal

- Making the Best of Tests and Procedures

- Staying Calm

- Getting Ready to Leave the Hospital

- Going Home

- Learning to Manage Medications at Home

- Summary

The Emergency Room Experience

You need to go to the emergency room (ER), or emergency department (ED), if you believe that you are at serious risk if you don't go. This can be a tough decision to make. Statistics show that only 5 percent of the people who go to emergency rooms are admitted to the hospital. As many as 90 percent of these people really should not have gone to the ER in the first place.

Call your doctor if you have time. Your doctor needs to know so that he can call the ER prior to your arrival if you want to have any hope of continuity of care and benefit from your physician's personal knowledge of you and your medical situation. Making this call is helpful to you, your doctor, and the ER doctor. Your doctor can also help you sort out whether an ER visit is necessary.

If you take many medications, it is helpful to keep that information and medical phone numbers on a card in your wallet. Let nurses, doctors, and other caregivers know that you have this information and where you have it.

Unlike restaurants and other businesses, emergency rooms don't necessarily treat you on a first-come-first-served basis. You do get in line and wait, but you may have to wait for an ER bed to become available or you may have to wait for people who are considered to have a more urgent crisis. Nurses "triage" patients, a screening upon admittance to the

ER to determine which patients need to be seen first. While sometimes inconvenient, the triaging process makes sense, especially if you put yourself in the shoes of the person who has an immediately life-threatening situation.

Another reason for waiting, after a decision has been made to admit you as an inpatient, may be that you need to wait for a hospital room or bed to become available. Carol has spent the night and part of the next day in the ER, making her room a draped off area in the ER and being served breakfast and lunch there before being wheeled to a real room. Using the ER for a temporary hospital bed is far from ideal, but "going with the flow" can be a big help as you endure situations like this.

It is crucial to have realistic expectations. You will probably receive care from good nurses and physicians but not your regular doctor. Most emergency room doctors have chosen to specialize in emergency medicine and completed specific education and experience requirements. ER doctors see a little bit of everything and encounter a wide array of accidents and diseases.

Experience has taught us to believe in what we call "Alice's Rule." Carol's mother used to say that you should expect your trip to the ER to take at least four hours from the time you leave your house until you return home. This rule was based on experience. We have seen little, if any, evidence in the past 20 years to argue with "Alice's Rule." You would be reasonable to expect to lose control of your situation, probably for the next four hours.

Communication is extremely important in part because the people working in the ER don't know you the way your regular doctor does. This adds a challenge to both you and the ER doctors in assuring that you receive the correct diagnosis and treatment. Generally, your ER doctor will contact your regular doctor while you are in the ER to keep your doctor informed and get input on your treatment. Be aware, though, that emergencies may happen; so be proactive. Talk to your doctor about how to handle one that arises. For example, you might ask whether and when to call the doctor at home.

You are likely to have x-rays and blood tests performed. Results generally are reported quickly for emergency room patients in order to get you home or to an area of the hospital that can take better care of your needs. Instead of waiting days for test results, you usually know results within an hour or two, often less.

If you have serious concern about a potentially life-threatening situation, you need to go to the ER. Having said that, know that once you start the process, it is very difficult to change the ER's mind or speed things up to get you home.

Before Going to the Hospital (Except in an Emergency)

Like any trip, a key to a positive hospital experience is preparation. One of the ways you can avoid many surprises and minimize your personal trauma involves doing your homework.

A first step is to check with your insurance company or your benefits department at work to make sure you understand your insurance benefits. Find out what advance notifications or approvals you need in the event of a non-emergency hospital admission. In Chapter Four, "Treating Medical Complications to Your Financial Health," we will cover insurance and financial issues in more depth. However, avoiding these surprises is important enough to warrant mention here.

Another important step is to find out as much as you can about the hospital where you are being admitted. You may have many questions to ask, including:

- Where is it?

- How do I get there?

- Where can my family park?

- Can they arrange for long-term parking?

- What are the visiting hours?

- Are private rooms available upon request, and if so how much is the additional cost?

Whether you are going as an inpatient or an outpatient, find out when you need to be there. If you are asked to be at the hospital at 5:00 A.M. for a 10:00 A.M. procedure, don't be afraid to ask "Do I really need to be there *that* early?" Chances are the answer is yes, but you will occasionally discover that there is a lot of cushion built into the time you are requested to arrive.

Also, find out where you should park and where you should go when you arrive at the hospital. Too many times, we have gone to the admitting department only to find out we needed to be at outpatient registration. We also have gone to a hospital's outpatient registration area, where they told us to go directly to the radiology department, which was more than a half-mile away!

Every hospital has its own unique set of operating procedures. We have found that even in the same hospital, different departments may have different registration procedures and locations. You may want to ask if a map or building layout is available, especially if you are going to a large hospital. Hospitals are often modern day mazes, the result of building additions over many years. In short, do everything you can in advance to avoid adding stress at the very beginning of your hospital experience with becoming lost or other snafus.

If you live alone or the people who live with you are traveling to be near you during your hospital stay, you will have to deal with many of the same issues you would deal with prior to going on vacation. When we recently traveled 2 1/2 hours upstate for several hospital stays, some of these issues we dealt with included stopping the mail and the newspaper, making arrangements for pets and canceling appointments. Unlike most vacations, medical trips often have an unknown return date, which further complicates planning. If you have children, the complexity becomes much greater.

When Eric was a small child, Carol was hospitalized many times. We had a standing invitation from both sets of grandparents to have him stay with them. This helped all of us through the uncertain transitions of moving in and out of the hospital.

What to Take to the Hospital

The short version of our advice is two words: pack light. You will not want to have so much with you that it becomes a worry or burden. Keep in mind that you may change rooms during your hospital stay. Many people will be coming and going from your room. While the vast majority of those people will be honest and trustworthy, and we have never lost anything in the hospital, you are still at risk of theft. In addition, your room will probably have very limited space. Last but not least, most hospital visits are short; most of your recuperation is likely to take place at home.

However, don't pack so lightly that you leave behind things that will make a big difference in your comfort during what you know will be a difficult experience, at least at times. Consider these essentials.

- **Writing supplies.** Take a pen or pencil and writing paper to jot things down to tell your doctors or nurses and to make notes about their instructions.

- **Spiritual materials.** Take spiritual, uplifting materials to read, such as a Bible and devotional readings. (You can also check with the chaplain's department to see what reading materials and other resources it has to offer.)

- **Reading material.** If you like to read, take a book or a few magazines with you. These can be left behind for future patients, if you wish.

- **Cash.** Take a few dollars, including a supply of change, which family members might occasionally find useful to make phone calls from pay phones. Take a list of phone numbers, too.

- **Pictures.** Consider taking a replaceable photograph or two and other reminders of home and family, especially if you will be far from home or anticipate a long stay.

- **Telephone calling card.** If you'll need to make long distance calls, make sure you know how you are going to do that. One option is a long distance calling card, some offering calls for 7 cents per minute or less. You might also ask if the hospital has an 800 line for out-of-town people to call patients.

- **Television schedule guide.** If you like to watch television, take a television schedule. Even though you generally won't have a full range of cable channels, the television is an important diversion for periods of boredom during your stay.

- **Cassette player.** Consider taking an inexpensive MP3, CD, or cassette player if you like to listen to music or books and expect to be in the hospital more than a day or two, recognizing that you are taking some risk of loss. Although conventional wisdom advises against bringing electronic devices to the hospital, we know that there are times when you don't feel like sitting up or focusing your eyes to read and there are many times when there is nothing worth watching on television. Music that is soothing to you can be very helpful in times of unusual stress.

- **Toiletries.** Take your own toothbrush, comb, and shaving supplies. If you like soft toilet paper or Kleenex, you will probably need to take your own!

- **Clothing.** Last but not least, take clothing! Hospital gowns, although sometimes necessary, leave a lot to be desired as a fashion statement and a lot exposed in the back! One time when Doug was hospitalized, Carol brought his sweatpants, walking shorts, and casual shirts for him to recover in style. He wasn't about to wear a hospital gown or pajamas.

Check (Some of) Your Dignity at the Door

Speaking of the silly hospital gowns, we need to say a few words about dignity and propriety. Robert Lipsyte shares a story describing the aftermath of his former wife eating too much cake at her birthday celebration during one of her hospital stays:

> (Margie) vomited neatly into a yellow plastic bucket. It was one chocolate splash. No big deal… (What) might have seemed odd or unpleasant, seemed natural, unnecessary for comment…. There is no Emily Post-Op to make hard and fast decisions about what is and isn't proper. (Robert Lipsyte, *In the Country of Illness: Comfort and Advice for the Journey*, New York: Knopf, 1998, p. 199.)

Carol chuckled when she read about Margie's incident. Carol remembers how hard she tried to convince her cardiologist that she was nauseated. Unable to convince the doctor that her nausea was brought on by the new medication he had prescribed, she eventually vomited all over her bed, the floor, and, yes, her cardiologist. (That convinced him!)

All celebrated people lose dignity on a close view.

– Napolean Bonaparte

Know Your Rights and Responsibilities

The American Hospital Association published a list of patient rights in 1973. AHA updated the Patient Bill of Rights in 1992, which can be accessed at www.aha.org. You probably won't have anyone read you your rights, but most hospitals have developed their own description of rights and responsibilities. They often make these resources available to patients when they are admitted.

Some of your most important rights as a patient include:

- The right to receive considerate and respectful care

- The right to be provided understandable information concerning diagnosis, treatment, and prognosis

- The right to make decisions about your plan of care

- The right to refuse a recommended treatment or plan of care

- The right to have an advance directive, such as a living will, healthcare proxy, or durable power of attorney for health care

- The right to consideration of your privacy

- The right to confidentiality regarding all communications

- The right to review your medical records pertaining to your medical care

- The right to ask and be informed of business relationships among the hospital, educational institutions, other healthcare providers, or payers that may influence your treatment and care

- The right to give your consent or decline to participate in proposed research studies or human experimentation

- The right to be informed of hospital policies and practices that relate to patient care, treatment, and responsibilities

Along with your rights go responsibilities. Many of your responsibilities are not only fairly obvious but are also in your best interest. We have already discussed several things you can do to make your interactions with the medical folks more effective. These include taking notes and making lists of your medical complaints and questions to ask (for each doctor if you are seeing more than one doctor). Very few patients want to be a pest, but don't hold back questions or symptoms because you are trying not to be a problem, either.

Finding the right balance between being assertive and being agreeable is every patient's unique responsibility. If you missed it, look again in Chapter Two in the section titled "Good Patient, Bad Patient."

What Should You Expect as an Inpatient?

This is really a trick question. There is no "typical day" in the life of a hospital inpatient. You can almost count on a few things, though.

> *Illness is a great leveler. At its touch, the artificial distinctions of society vanish away. People in a hospital are just people.*
>
> – M. Thorek

You will probably find it noisy. Sleep difficulties are common. Interruptions will occur when you are sleeping. You may be awakened early in the morning, perhaps unintentionally. The night shift's last job before leaving seems to be irritating and arousing patients with seemingly trivial sleep interruptions, such as putting fresh ice water, sheets and towels in patient rooms.

Medications will be delivered to your room and served to you. While you are in the hospital, you have a limited role in managing medications. You will generally be told not to bring medications to the hospital. When your history and physical examination is done, you will be asked to list the medications you normally take, the dosages, the times per day you take the medication, and other relevant information. During your stay, your nurses will deliver medications to your bedside. You need only to question the nurse if it seems like something is out of line. Carol adds that she always counts her pills, just like at home, and notices when something looks different. If something looks different, such as different color or size, it might be a generic substitute. We strongly recommend asking the nurse to make sure the medications are correct.

Something else you can expect, if your doctor has ordered laboratory tests, is a visit from the phlebotomist or lab technician (those are the Medi-speak words for vampire) before your breakfast is served.

The next thing to look forward to might be breakfast in bed. Don't get too excited. After the early morning visits by the phlebotomist and the linenologist, the next really exciting event isn't likely to occur until 7:30 or 8:00 A.M., maybe even later, when breakfast arrives. Lunch and dinner will also be delivered to your bed. You will have some choice in your meal selection although your first few meals will probably be selected for

> *Hospital rooms seem to have vastly more ceiling than any rooms people live in.*
>
> – Bertha Damon

you. When you select food from a menu, you can generally order more than one beverage, vegetables, or bread item. This is useful as a way to hedge against some part of your meal not appealing to you. Your food may not taste good, because it doesn't taste good, or because it is a meal which your stomach does not feel ready for. Food may not taste good because your appetite is affected by being sick. Your food will be reasonably nutritious, not necessarily heart-healthy unless a special diet is prescribed, and rarely gourmet-style cuisine. Doug's favorite hospital foods are macaroni and cheese, jello, and vanilla pudding. Unfortunately, you can't get all of these favorites every meal, but you can always ask!

Doctors will visit you but scheduled arrivals at your room are rare. Some doctors make their rounds to see their patients in the hospital early, before going to their office, which might mean you are awakened fairly early. Other doctors come at the end of their day, which can tend to make you anxious if you are waiting for test results or a medical decision. If you are not a "morning person," an early morning doctor's visit may come at a time when you are not very awake. Keeping a running journal or questions and complaints list can be very helpful, particularly as an early morning aid during your doctor's bedside visit. It helps also to tell your nurse what questions you have so that he or she can be your memory advocate. Nurses have jotted notes on the front of Carol's chart from time to time to remind doctors of a new symptom or other important information.

You will probably see many doctors you have never seen before, including your doctor's partners or associates and other specialists. Many larger hospitals participate in teaching programs for physicians and other medical professionals. In these hospitals you are likely to see interns and residents. They will ask you many questions. You may feel like you answer the same questions over and over again. You probably will. Carol had an interesting experience during her first hospital stay in January, 1979. Doctors would walk into her room with as many as eight residents. She was a young patient with an unusual condition, so she was asked a lot of questions. She knew that she had the right not to answer all the questions from interns and residents, but she felt that it was useful and helpful and did not mind.

Interns and residents often serve as right-hand assistants to your physicians. They can also be an advocate for you and provide more extensive explanations to you than your attending physician. But don't be alarmed if an intern, resident, or post-graduate fellow makes a discovery from your x-rays or lab tests that is a significant departure from what you've heard from your physician. It is common for an intern to think he or she has made a wonderful discovery, and then proceed to share this information with a patient before talking to the attending physician.

Doug recalls an unfortunate situation along these lines, which he describes below.

> I remember an incident about ten years ago. A post-graduate "fellow" saw Carol during a hospitalization for heart arrhythmia. The fellow was brand new to her case although he was with a group which had helped care for her for close to ten years. He "saw something" on an electrocardiogram that he believed was a problem. More significantly, he then decided to share this news with Carol and me. We found the news quite alarming. We fretted overnight. The next day we asked her cardiologist about this news. He dismissed the "new finding" and assured us that there was no significant change in her electrocardiogram and no change in treatment was called for.

What's the moral of the story? Don't assume that the intern, resident or fellow is correct. No one needs to have a sleepless night, much less when you're in the hospital and even less because of a comment by an inexperienced doctor who knows very little about your medical history.

Visitors

As a patient you can expect to have too many visitors, not enough visitors, or visitors at the wrong times. Most patients love to have visitors, who often bring an emotional boost not only for the patient but also for the patient's immediate family and primary support givers. One memorable example for us is when Carol's friends once came to wash and curl her hair after she had been in the hospital for two weeks and not allowed to take a shower. However, there are times when patients don't feel like talking to or seeing anyone. Some visitors stay too long. Some visitors talk too loud, ask too many questions, or offer too much advice and opinion. Knowing how and when to put limits on visitors is key.

If people ask about visiting you or a family member, suggest that they call first to ask. Your need and readiness for visitors may change daily, if not more often. Doug once visited a friend who was in the final stages of cancer. Doug had called a few days earlier to ask if his friend would like a visitor. The friend had said, "No, it's not a good day." When Doug arrived at the friend's house a few days later (after calling to see if it was a good time for him to come), the first thing his friend did was apologize for telling Doug not to visit earlier in the week. Doug said, "You were smart," which surprised his friend. From his personal experience, Doug knew that there are times when "just say no" is the best advice for handling visitors, which is essentially just being honest.

If all else fails, you can put a "No Visitors" or "Visitors Inquire at Nurses Station" sign on the door to your room. There is a good chance that one of your nurses will be kind enough to put up such a sign and make it look official!

Now that we have attacked visitors, let us reassert the importance of visitors as a connection to a patient's world and life outside the hospital. Visitors are an essential part of the patient's team. We offer a few helpful tips for visitors.

- **Listen to the patient.** Remember that very few of the many people the patient will encounter during the stay are friends or family. Most people just appreciate being listened to. One helpful reminder is that God gave you two ears and one mouth for a reason, suggesting that you use your ears twice as much as your mouth.

- **Offer support.** Patients need support, not opinions or judgment. This is a corollary to the first suggestion.

- **Suggest how you can help.** Suggest practical things you can do. You may see little things to do for the patient, such as watering her flowers, combing her hair, getting her a cool drink, or washing her hair. Perhaps there are tasks at home that you can help take care of.

- **Be sensitive.** Visitors need to be sensitive to the patient's situation and mood. We once had a visitor just a few minutes before a delicate, dangerous procedure was to be performed. The visitor totally missed the seriousness of the situation. He was very loud and boisterous, full of inappropriate humor, and had an energy level totally out of proportion to where the patient and family were.

- **Respect the roommate.** Be respectful of the patient's roommate. Don't be too noisy. Appreciate that the roommate may have an even more serious or difficult situation than your friend. Or maybe they are having a bad day.

- **Don't stay too long.** Many patients would find it difficult to tell you to leave. Generally, staying no more than 10 or 15 minutes is a good guideline.

- **Touch the patient.** If appropriate to the patient's personality and your relationship with the patient, touch can very powerful. Holding someone's hand at a time that they are confronting uncertainty and fear, separation from the family and "normal life" can be very helpful. Carol remembers her mother's gentle touch to her forehead as being very helpful in a very stressful emergency. During another dangerous procedure, Doug stood at the foot of Carol's bed and held her toes. For Carol, this special touch was comforting.

Humor Helps You Heal

Humor is an indispensable aid to health and healing. There are books full of humor related to hospitals and doctors. They illustrate one type of humor. The other type of humor is seeing the humorous in the midst of your own serious situation. As one source of humor, consider the following list of medical terminology. See what terms you can add to the list. We would love to hear your nominations at our Web site, www.patientpress.com. See Chapter Nine, "Realigning Your Attitude," for more on the power of humor.

Uncommon Medical Terminology

Term	Definition
Artery	The study of fine paintings
Barium	What you do after CPR fails
Benign	What you are after you be eight
Colic	A sheep dog
Coma	A punctuation mark
GI series	Baseball game between soldiers
Medical staff	A doctor's cane
Morbid	A higher offer
Nitrate	Lower than the day rate
Node	Was aware of
Organic	Church musician
Outpatient	A person who has fainted
Post operative	A letter carrier
Rectum	Damn near killed 'em
Seizure	Roman emperor
Serology	Study of English knighthood
Tumor	An extra pair
Vein	Conceited
Varicose veins	Veins which are close together

Making the Best of Tests and Procedures

You can probably count on being stuck, stabbed, and probed with needles and other medical devices during your stay, so we have included some insights we have had regarding the challenges of tests and medical procedures.

They do certainly give very strange, and newfangled, names to diseases.

— Plato

First, be sure that you understand and exercise your right to know why you are having a test performed. If you've had the same procedure recently, ask why you need to have the test repeated. Often, previous test results and x-rays can be forwarded and even faxed to your doctor or to the hospital.

You also have the right to be treated politely and with respect. Learn as much as you want to learn, and develop as positive an attitude as possible. If you have fears, name them and discuss them with whomever you know who will listen without judging or trying to take over and "fix" the problems. Having a positive attitude does not mean that you need to act like you're not afraid or free of concerns.

If you are having a test, procedure or operation performed the next day, your nurse may tell you that you are NPO. Don't be offended. You are not being insulted. NPO stands for "non per os," which is Latin for "nothing by mouth." Generally, you will be NPO after midnight, meaning that you cannot eat or drink after that time until after your procedure. Medications, taken with a small sip of water, are generally exceptions.

Try to remember that nobody is perfect. You may have breakfast delivered to you even though you think that you are NPO. If you think you are not supposed to eat breakfast but have breakfast delivered to you, don't just assume you can eat breakfast. Call your nurse. Make sure that your test is still scheduled. If it is, have your food removed until after your test. Otherwise, you are likely to cause a delay in your diagnosis and treatment, and possibly extend your hospital stay.

Staying Calm

Sometimes it is hard to maintain your sense of humor when you are placed in especially stressful situations. Nonetheless, our best advice is to try to stay calm. For Doug, this has sometimes been a case of "do as I say, not as I do," as he describes below.

I remember being anything but calm when I was undergoing one of the pre-surgical procedures. I haven't always been a poster child for good attitude. I remember when I had an angiogram (a heart catheterization procedure) which my surgeon needed to show him a "blueprint" of the area he would be operating, prior to surgery on my pituitary gland in 1991. That was a very stressful experience. It was the first invasive procedure I would experience. I also knew that it was just the beginning of a lot of invasions into my body. I was apprehensive and scared.

Because I was apprehensive, I was also tense. When the radiologist had difficulty finding the artery he needed, I got even more tense, which made the doctor's job that much harder. Trying to help, one of the medical technicians offered me some totally useless advice, which actually came across as more of a scolding: "This would be a lot easier if you would just relax."

I wanted to respond: "No #@&@#, Sherlock. Thank you for that incredible insight. Don't you think I know that? I'd love to relax. But at the moment, I've got needles and catheters in various places. I'm lying here pretty exposed on a hard, cold, white table. This isn't going smoothly and I still have surgery on a still unidentified glob in the middle of my head awaiting me. Plus there's this genius telling me to relax. Right now I am finding that very difficult to accomplish."

I didn't say it but I almost wish I had. That was sure how I was feeling at that moment.

As Doug demonstrated, "just relax" is not a natural response. Our ancestors relied upon a hard-wired, fine-tuned system to identify and respond to frequent threats upon their lives. Human beings still carry this response with them into every stressful situation. Today, health professionals call this the "fight-or-flight response." When you perceive that you are being threatened, the stress causes your entire musculoskeletal system to become rigid. (The fight-or-flight response is discussed in more detail in Chapter Six, "Understanding Your Mind-Body Connection.")

While the fight-or-flight response was absolutely essential when our ancestors were under attack from saber-tooth tigers and other beasts, it is just about the last thing you need when you are about to undergo medical testing.

Research showing the dramatic impact of relaxation on the healing process is exploding. There is scientific backing and documentation of what common sense has told us for years. If you'd like to learn more about this exciting area, read the newest edition of one of the first books written on this topic, *The Relaxation Response* (Herbert Benson, M.D., New York: Avon, 2000). Another resource you might look for is *The Relaxation and Stress Reduction Workbook* (Martha Davis, Ph.D., Elizabeth Robbins Eshelman, M.S.W., and Matthew McKay, Ph.D., New York: New Harbinger, 1995).

As much as Doug didn't appreciate the advice he received ("This would be a lot easier if you would just relax."), in reality, you can stay calm even under difficult circumstances. You have the ability to relax if you have the knowledge and skills. You just need to know how.

Harvard Medical School's Mind/Body Medical Institute recommends what they call "mini" relaxation techniques. "Minis" focus on breathing techniques to help reduce anxiety and tension. This technique relies upon diaphragmatic breathing, where your stomach rises about an inch as you breathe in and falls as you breathe out.

Here's one example. Count slowly up to four. As you exhale, count slowly back down to one. As you inhale, say "1-2-3-4" and as you exhale say "4-3-2-1." Repeat this exercise several times. This technique will help you relax in heavy traffic, in a tense meeting, or while you are apprehensively waiting for a medical test.

The Mind/Body Medical Institute says "the only time minis don't work is when you forget to do them." So try one, now or any time. They are free and have no negative side effects. When have you been offered such a great prescription?

The mind-body connection, relaxation response, relaxation techniques, minis and other key coping skills are covered in Chapter Six.

Getting Ready to Leave the Hospital

There are a few similarities between the process of being discharged (released) from the hospital and checking out of a hotel. However, you probably won't receive an itemized statement or be able to view it on your television screen.

If you can, find out in advance which doctor will be discharging you. We have experienced times when only one doctor has the final "authority" to release you from the hospital. Also, find out when you will be discharged, including approximate time of day. This has become more difficult to determine since it has become almost as common for patients to be released in the evening as any other time of day.

It is also critical to make sure that you receive clear instructions from your doctors as well as the nurse who is discharging you. Key considerations are guidance for when to see your doctor for follow-up, what events should trigger a call to your doctor, which medications to take, instructions on how and when to take them, any other treatment instructions, and any restrictions on your activities. If you are up to the task, take notes or have the person driving you home take notes. You may even consider tape recording the instructions. The last minute barrage of information can be overwhelming, particularly when you are eager to get out the hospital door.

Going Home

As we have said before, have reasonable expectations. Sometimes a medical crisis makes it very obvious that you need to go to the hospital for diagnosis and treatment. When you leave the hospital, it is natural to expect that you will feel better and have solved a problem. Unfortunately, sometimes your stay in the hospital consists of a battery of tests, often inconclusive or simply ruling out specific causes, and answers are still incomplete when you leave.

We have felt at times that we were going home not because we were better or that a mystery had been solved, but that we and our doctors had run out of meaningful tests to perform. If this happens, the end of your hospital stay may feel anticlimactic. Sometimes you reach an impasse. Try to accept the fact that you haven't solved the problem that took you to the hospital in the first place. We have experienced this feeling on numerous occasions as Carol left the hospital. She wasn't well, or even fully diagnosed, but there really wasn't any reason to keep her in the hospital. It was a very unsettling experience to leave the hospital without the answers we had hoped for.

Learning to Manage Medications at Home

While you are in the hospital, you have a limited role in managing medications. This situation changes dramatically when you go home, where managing your medications can be a significant challenge. This is true especially if you take more than two or three pills daily. After many years of taking a variety of medications, we still forget occasionally to take a pill. The task becomes more difficult as the number of medications you take increases, as your health condition worsens, or when temporary illnesses compound your mix of medications. You may need a system. We both did!

We can offer some practical suggestions for managing medications at home. Go to your pharmacy and buy a pill container, which you can fill daily, weekly, or as often as you need to. Most people can use a weekly container with compartments for each day of the week. Using one of these containers, you can go through a weekly routine, putting all of your medications for the week in the container. Carol has three weekly containers. Each contains the medications she must take at a specific time of day. For instance, her eight pills she takes before breakfast are in one container. If she wonders if she forgot her morning medications, all she needs to do is check the daily spot in the morning container.

Another approach is to put medicine in cups once a day for your various doses. Then if you think you forgot a dose, all you have to do is check the cup. Remembering whether or not you've taken a particular pill is another brainteaser, especially if you sometimes find yourself in a room in your home and can't remember why you went there, as we often do!

Remembering to take medications is a common everyday challenge. Setting an alarm clock or a watch alarm is a practical way to remember to take medications. Many people find it useful to list their medications and dosages on an index card. (You can put the card in your wallet for use by medical professionals in an emergency situation.) Some people check off medications as they take them, a particularly good idea if you have problems with memory. Some medications should be taken with food, while others should not be taken with food. Some don't matter. So it makes sense to read the instructions and talk to your pharmacist if you have questions about your regime. We have found our pharmacist to be a very valuable resource.

If you need to administer injections at home and have trouble remembering whether or not you've taken a dose, you might set out your needles or syringes for the day. When Doug has used a needle, he replaces the orange protector but not the cap at the other end. Then he disposes the needle in a container designed for that purpose. But if he forgets to dispose of the needle immediately, by not having replaced the cap, he makes sure that he never accidentally reuses a needle after getting distracted or interrupted.

Some medications require a strict time regimen. Don't be afraid to ask your doctor or pharmacist just how strictly you need to follow the suggested time intervals between dosages of your medications. If you have some flexibility on timing, it might make it easier to remember when to take medications. For example, you might take one of each pill when you wake up in the morning. Some pills might be taken once, twice, or three or more times per day. If you take six or eight medications, all on different schedules, life can be pretty complicated. If you find out that you have some flexibility on timing, you may be able to take several pills at the same time, at lunch or mid-afternoon, rather than having a pill to take every hour on the hour. However, the instructions are extremely important for some medications, so take time to ask the trained professionals for their advice.

If you are new to the world of illness, beware of your possible emotional reaction to taking a variety of medications. Everybody is different. Doug has struggled with this issue much more than Carol, who has pretty much accepted the fact that she needs to take a variety of medications daily and is grateful for the medications to improve her quality of life and keep her alive. We strongly recommend you adopt Carol's accepting attitude toward medications. Doug knows intellectually that he needs to take nine or ten different prescription medications and that it has nothing to do with his self-worth or his value as a human being. But he still has to wrestle with emotions that range from embarrassment to inadequacy.

Summary

Like many aspects of life with your illness, dealing with hospitals, enduring diagnostic and therapeutic treatment, and managing your medications aren't always fun. Knowing what to expect, including the unexpected, and learning to relax under pressure can reap major benefits for you and make the hospital experience as pleasant as possible. Expecting surprises, maintaining your sense of humor, and learning relaxation techniques are also important.

The next chapter focuses on treatment of medical complications to your financial situation, in hopes of making that part of your experience as good as possible, too.

There is no Emily Post-Op to make hard and fast decisions about what is and isn't proper.

– Robert Lipsyte

FOUR

Treating Medical Complications to Your Financial Health

Hospital gowns are like the cheapest HMO
option: you only think you're covered.

– Anonymous

When you are a hospital inpatient, one of your primary goals is to leave the hospital and return home. Unfortunately, the financial impact of your hospital stay lives long beyond your stay. In many ways, going home means that the financial challenges have just begun.

Because there are far too many complex issues and topics for us to cover this topic thoroughly in one chapter, this chapter covers the main points and provides useful resources. Those resources include entire books devoted to many of the individual topics which we will cruise through in this chapter.

This chapter focuses on complications to your life that result from the financial side of your encounters with doctors, hospitals, and other medical providers. The chapter is organized around the following headings:

- General Advice

- This May Feel Like a Car Accident

- Why Does Everything Cost So Much?

- Understanding the Lingo

- Who Pays?

- Understanding Your Coverage

- Medicare

- Key Decisions

- Filing Claims

- Treating Complications

- Dealing with the Collection Process

- Summary

General Advice

First of all, have reasonable expectations. Hope for the best but expect surprises. Maybe even expect Murphy's law ("if anything can go wrong, it will") to apply in all situations. When things go wrong, stay as calm as possible. For example, don't overreact when you get threatening letters or phone calls regarding outstanding bills for healthcare services. Having a sense of humor is especially useful. Things probably are not going to be as bad as we have made it sound—at least not most of the time—but it does pay to take things in stride.

This May Feel Like a Car Accident

When Doug was asked if he felt like he had been run over by a car after his surgery, he responded, "I feel like I've been run over by a truck." It's ironic that he was asked that question because it turns out there are some interesting parallels and contrasts between medical cost and insurance benefits and car insurance.

If you are familiar with what happens from the time you have a car accident until the insurance company pays the claim, you will not be surprised when you deal with some of the financial aspects of healthcare services. Consider the following comparison table (continued on the next page), which illustrates some of these parallels.

When you're involved in a car accident...	When you're involved in a healthcare crisis...
• You made critical choices about coverage before your collision.	• You made critical choices about medical coverage before you got sick.
• When the accident happens, you are concerned about personal injuries, hoping none are serious.	• In the hospital, you are concerned about getting the right treatment and getting well.
• Then you begin to wonder about damage to your car and insurance coverage.	• Then you begin to wonder about the adequacy of your insurance coverage.

When you're involved in a car accident...	When you're involved in a healthcare crisis...
• You wonder how much is covered, whose policy will pay, how to file a claim and where and how to get an estimate.	• You wonder how much is covered, whose policy will pay, how to file a claim, and where and how to get answers.
• Everything seems to cost double or triple the amount you expected.	• Everything seems to cost double or triple the amount you expected.
• Sometimes your insurance company resists approving or paying your claim.	• Sometimes your insurance company resists approving or paying your claims.
• Many of the terms confuse you, like deductibles and subrogation.	• Many of the terms confuse like deductibles, co-payments, contractual adjustments, provider network, pre-certification, and authorization.

Why Does Everything Cost So Much?

Healthcare services make up almost one-sixth of the U.S. economy. Since the mid-1960s there has been an unusual market dynamic at work; that is, consumers of healthcare services generally do not pay directly for services they consume. They pay, but not directly. Instead, they pay for healthcare services through their insurance premiums, their taxes to finance Medicaid and other federal and state programs, and in the cost of products they purchase because manufacturers pass on costs of healthcare benefits to their customers.

Many patients pay for part of their healthcare services, but what individual patients pay has very little to do with the services they consume. This dynamic is compounded by the explosion of new technology in the second half of the 20th

> A hospital bed is a parked taxi with the meter running.
>
> – Groucho Marx

century, which has come at an incredible financial cost.

As a result of many factors, healthcare services are costly to provide and expensive to purchase. Some services seem especially expensive because some procedures are marked up a higher percentage than other procedures. Hospitals legitimately have a profit margin on such procedures, which sometimes helps them to offset the losses that they sustain on many other services, including services provided disproportionately to patients covered by governmental programs, who often pay hospitals less than half of the cost for some services.

For the most part, you should take extreme stories of high-priced procedures with a grain of salt. Much like the stories of toilet seats and nuts and bolts that supposedly cost the Defense Department several hundred dollars, the real picture can get distorted. It is also important to know that if every payer paid the full price, the full price would be much lower than it is.

Physicians' services sometimes seem to be overly expensive, but there is often a reasonable explanation. Many insurance plans limit payment to the physician's standard charge for a procedure, or some percentage of that charge. Therefore, physicians sometimes feel that they need to keep their prices higher or else risk shortchanging themselves by dragging down the amount calculated by the insurance company.

Although we don't feel particularly comfortable negotiating prices, when we had an experience where the bill for surgical services exceeded what insurance paid, we simply asked to pay the amount over several months. The physician responded by writing off the difference and explained his rationale, similar to the one described above.

Understanding the Lingo

Like any other specialized field, healthcare finance has its own language. We've highlighted in bold font (**bold font**) terms and phrases that may be unfamiliar to you. The terms highlighted are defined in the glossary below. Other terms are also included in the glossary.

Brief Glossary of Medical Financial Jargon

Contractual adjustments. The difference between the amount of the provider's standard charges and the amount the provider agreed to accept as payment in full.

Co-payment. Portion of charges that patient must pay after satisfying the deductible amount. Commonly, the co-pay percentage is 10 to 20 percent, subject to an annual maximum that varies by policy.

Credentialing. Obtaining and reviewing the documentation of professional providers. Generally includes reviewing information provided by the provider and verifying that the information is correct and complete.

Deductibles. Amount that patient must pay before insurance coverage begins to pay for services.

Explanation of benefits (EOB). Statement that insurance plan or HMO sends to the patient, explaining the amount and basis for payment to doctors, hospitals and other providers, or to the patient.

Health maintenance organization (HMO). A legal corporation that offers health insurance and medical care. HMOs provide a range of comprehensive healthcare services for a specified group at a fixed periodic rate.

Managed care. A system of providing healthcare through which access, cost, and quality are controlled by direct interventions before, during, or after service delivery. Plans use a variety of techniques, such as utilization review, quality assurance programs, and pre-admission certification to better manage the care delivered.

Primary coverage. The insurance coverage that providers should first bill medical claims.

Provider. Whoever provides healthcare, including doctors, therapists, nurse-practitioners, hospitals and others who provide or deliver healthcare.

Provider network. Providers who your insurance plan recognizes as eligible to serve you and be compensated by the plan.

Secondary coverage. The insurance coverage that providers should bill claims after the primary coverage has determined the amount it will cover. Secondary coverage usually takes into account the payments made by the primary plan.

Traditional indemnity plan. "Old-fashioned" insurance plan that covers virtually all services and generally pays a provider what the provider establishes as its usual and customary charges.

Utilization review. Method used by some insurers and employers to identify and reduce inappropriate and unnecessary care.

Who Pays?

First, we need to acknowledge that not everyone has adequate health insurance coverage. If you don't have insurance, there may be resources available in your community to help you pay for healthcare services. Your hospital may have a foundation or other organization to help patients who do not have the economic ability to pay their bills. Even if such help is available, you face a tremendous financial and emotional challenge.

Even for people fortunate enough to have insurance coverage, there are no easy answers, but there are some general rules.

- Beware, there are exceptions to every rule.

- Medicare is responsible for *most* of the cost of your care if you are over 65 or disabled.

- Insurance coverage should fill in the gap for services not covered by Medicare. Many people covered by Medicare purchase private insurance, called Medi-gap insurance.

- If you're under 65, your benefits depend on choices you made before you needed care. If you anticipated the real possibility of needing healthcare services some time down the road, you probably purchased, with the help of your employer, insurance or health maintenance organization (HMO) coverage.

> God heals and the doctor takes the fee.
>
> – Benjamin Franklin

You should expect to receive bills from the hospital and from each doctor you see. You often will get two or more bills for the same procedure, one bill from the doctor who performed the procedure and one from the facility (such as hospital or surgery center) where your procedure was performed. You may also get bills from other healthcare professionals that you may not have seen, such as radiologists and anesthesiologists.

If you find all of this confusing, take comfort in knowing you are not alone. Even after more than 20 years of trying to manage this aspect of life-changing illness, we get confused and have difficulty keeping track of things.

Understanding Your Coverage

You probably made healthcare coverage choices long before your current crisis. You may also have some latitude to change some components of your choice annually, during your insurance plan's enrollment period. Once you are in the midst of heavy consumption of medical services, you need to accept your coverage as it is, for the most part. Read your policies if you can make sense of them. Read your employer's information, which may be more user friendly, or ask your company's employee benefits department to assist you.

Prior authorization or pre-certification has become very common. These terms essentially mean that you need to get the insurance company's approval of services in advance. Even many traditional indemnity plans have authorization and certification rules that just a few years ago were limited to HMOs and other **managed care** plans. These policies can be very frustrating and time-consuming. They often cause delays in receiving services. Sometimes it may look as if your plan is delaying or avoiding an expensive procedure. Do not be afraid to ask and continue to ask why there are delays or why you're not getting answers.

Medicare

If you have Medicare coverage, you will face most of the same issues as with private insurance. You have an advantage in that 40 million people are covered by Medicare. As a result, there are many independent and government publications to help you navigate through one of the U.S. Government's largest and most complicated programs.

Medicare is an extremely complicated topic. We will barely be able to put a dent in this diverse topic in this chapter. Here are some main points about Medicare:

- Most recipients are covered by Medicare Part A, which includes coverage for inpatient hospital services.

- In 2000, the Medicare Part A annual **deductible** was $776. **Co-payments** were $194 per day for the 61st through 90th day of a prolonged hospital stay and $388 per day for the 91st through 150th days.

- Physician services and many outpatient services are covered under Medicare's Part B program, which is not automatically provided to Part A beneficiaries. Part B requires a premium payment ($45.50 per month in 2000). The Part B premium is generally deducted from Social Security recipients' monthly checks.

Deductibles and co-payment amounts are adjusted annually to reflect changes in the cost of living.

The Official U.S. Government Web site for Medicare Information is an excellent source of information to guide you in dealing with Medicare issues. The address is www.medicare.gov. There is a handbook at this site, called "Medicare and You 2000."

Key Decisions

Decisions that you make long before your medical crisis or hospital stay determine the type and amount of coverage and benefits available to you.

Most employer-based health plans give a range of options, including a **traditional indemnity plan** and a **health maintenance organization** (HMO). Sometimes these options have very different levels of premiums and annual **deductibles**. All other things being equal, the higher your annual deductible, the lower the annual premium. Likewise, all other things being equal, the higher your **co-payment percentage**, the lower your annual premium. Some options offer you a choice of annual deductible.

In general, you buy insurance to protect you against the unknown; you share the risk with your insurance company and millions of other policyholders. You may know enough about your medical situation to know that your costs of medical care are going to be substantial. Based on this knowledge, you can make some assumptions and do some calculations to help you determine which option to select.

We will use our personal situation as an example. We know we are going to have high medical costs every year. Doug's doctor prescribes injections, which we must order through our pharmacist. Together with conventional medications, our monthly costs exceed $1,500 for prescriptions alone. For example, let's say that we estimate our total cost for the year to be $20,000, including prescriptions and doctor visits.

Assume that we have two health insurance options to choose from. Option 1 costs $6,000 per year and Option 2 costs $4,800 per year. Both options have a deductible, meaning we have to pay for all services until the year-to-date costs reach the amount of the deductible. With Option 1, the deductible is $200, so the insurance company would start paying claims after the first $200. Option 2 has a $1,000 deductible, which sounds like a lot of cost to pick up. But there's more to consider. Both options have a 10 percent co-payment percentage, meaning that after we have reached the deductible of $200 or $1,000, the insurance company pays 90 percent and we pay 10 percent. Both options also have an annual maximum of $2,500 on the total deductibles and co-payments we are responsible to pay.

Let's see how the math works out.

			Option 1	Option 2
Total medical bills	1		$20,000	$20,000
Annual premium	2		$6,000	$4,800
Annual deductible	3		$200	$1,000
Co-payment percentage	4		10%	10%
Co-payments	5	Line 4 times (Line 1 minus Line 3)	$1,980	$1,900
Out-of-pocket costs	6	Note	$2,180	$2,500
Out-of-pocket costs plus premiums	7	Line 2 plus Line 6	$8,180	$7,300

Note—Lesser of $2,500 (maximum out-of-pocket) or sum of lines 3 and 5.

With Option 1, we would pay an annual premium of $6,000 plus deductibles and co-payments of $2,180, for a total of $8,180. If we select Option 2, we would pay a premium of $4,800 plus out-of-pocket expenses at the maximum of $2,500, for a total of $7,300. What may have looked at first glance like the more expensive option, having to pick up the first $1,000 of medical bills, turns out to be less expensive.

The cost comparison table above is just one illustration of some of the wrinkles you need to watch out for as you make these choices in the future. You also need to consider whether you have the full choice of doctors, hospitals and types of care that you would like to have. Otherwise, you may need to pay out of your pocket for services that your insurance coverage excludes.

Your coverage options probably also challenge you to make a decision regarding how much freedom you have in selecting your primary physician and specialists, or which hospitals and outpatient centers you can use. Your coverage options also include how stringent the prior approval process is.

Filing Claims

Dr. Albert Einstein once said that even he couldn't understand the federal tax code. He would probably have been similarly confused if he had to file insurance claim forms. Submitting claims for medical benefits can certainly be a hair-raising experience, even for an Einstein.

If you are working and your coverage is through an employer-sponsored health plan, your employee benefits department will be your source for claims forms and one of your primary sources of information. Depending on our current insurance carrier and the policy of the doctor, we have had experiences ranging from filing our own claims for most of our doctor visits and prescriptions to having the healthcare providers submit most of the claims. Even though it may seem that you lose control by having the providers do the paper work, it is really a blessing. You will still have plenty of work to do to manage the bills you receive and the **explanation of benefits** reports that you receive from payers.

As mentioned above, if the doctor's office is willing to bill insurance on your behalf, let them. They generally have expertise about how to fill out the forms correctly. Sometimes they also have the expertise to help break "logjams" that sometimes occur in getting a claim processed. Here are some tips to make the claims filing process smoother.

- Make sure that your doctor is part of the **provider network** if your coverage limits your choice of physician. Understand the coverage implications if he or she is not part of the network.

- Make sure you have satisfied any requirements to have services approved in advance.

- Make sure you have the most current insurance card and the correct address and phone numbers.

- Have your doctor's office make a copy of your insurance card (they will generally ask you for one).

- If you are covered by more than one insurance plan (for example, both you and your spouse are employed and are covered by each spouse's policy), make sure you know which one is **primary** and which one is **secondary**. Make sure that this is clear to your doctor's office staff.

- Keep track of the status of each claim if you have the patience to do so.

Treating Complications

Often, for a variety of reasons, there is a long delay in payment by your insurance company. This is complicated further when one or more of the following occurs.

- You are covered by more than one policy (such as your policy and your spouse's policy) and the primary payer is challenging whether it should be the primary payer rather than the secondary payer.

- You, your doctor, or the hospital didn't properly determine that you were covered prior to receiving your treatment.

- You, your doctor, or the hospital didn't bill the insurance company properly.

- Stuff happens. Sometimes there seems to be no apparent reason for delays. Whether it is "something falling into a crack" or "stuck in somebody's in-basket," delays sometimes just happen.

Here are several suggestions for treating these complications.

- Find out why there is a delay.

- Start by calling your insurance company.

- Take notes and keep your information well organized.

- Write down:
  - Name of the person you talked to
  - Date of your call and the person's phone number
  - What they told you was the reason for the delay
  - How and when the claim will be resolved

- File your notes in a place where you can easily find them.

- Don't be afraid to ask for help. If you have trouble finding out why there is a delay or if you find out that your claim has been or will be denied, ask your doctor's office or the business office of your hospital to work with you to get the insurance company's cooperation.

Remember that there is almost always a higher authority to appeal to. If you can't get satisfaction, ask for the supervisor of the person you are talking to. If necessary, go to the vice president or even the president of the hospital or insurance plan. Try to keep from getting too discouraged by this process, which can sometimes seem insane.

Dealing with the Collection Process

We were shocked the first time we received a collection notice. We were in our early twenties, proud of our credit record and terrified that it might be marred. Since then, we have gotten a handful of collection notices, all related to medical services. We are no longer shocked.

Sometimes an unpaid bill will be turned over to the collection agency a very short time after you received a totally nonthreatening hospital bill. Perhaps you were led to believe that the insurance company was planning to pay the bill. Don't get too excited.

Usually these matters can get resolved, short of you having a blemish on your credit record. Start by calling the agency and register your surprise that the bill has been referred to them and indicate that you have been fully cooperating with the hospital in getting the bill paid.

Next, call the hospital and insist on speaking to the director of patient financial services, business office manager, or similar person. Express your dissatisfaction with the fact that your account has been turned over to collection and refer to your notes of earlier conversations with the hospital and the insurance company. If there is something the hospital still hasn't done that the insurance company requested, urge them to do it. Insurance companies seem to have an insatiable desire for documentation.

Call the insurance company yourself to see what the problem is. If necessary, go to the top of the organization. Sometimes persistence makes the difference in whether or not services are covered. When all else fails, consider writing a letter. After several months of "getting nowhere" with convincing a hospital to bill the right insurance company for medical tests for Carol, Doug wrote the following note to the hospital:

Dear Sir or Madam,

For the umpteenth time, our insurance is (insurance company, address, and telephone number). Please quit sending us these notices. Everyone else gets paid timely by (insurance company) so you must be billing something incorrectly. Please quit bothering us with these notices.

Sincerely,

Doug Langenfeld

The matter was resolved fairly quickly.

Usually, your insurance company will pay for most of your care. Often, even if the insurance company pays less than the full amount charged by the hospital, the hospital voluntarily or involuntarily writes of all or part of the balance. If there is some amount still due to the hospital after all insurance payments and adjustments, most hospitals will work out payment terms that are fairly liberal.

In any of these dealings, keeping good records of written and oral communications is essential. And whenever you start to doubt whether your rights are being respected, consider consulting an attorney.

Summary

The financial side of health care is complex, confusing, and constantly changing. When you are dealing with serious medical and other life-changing issues, the additional weight of financial complications can be very stressful.

This chapter has offered an overview of the financial side of health care, suggested other resources to help you explore these issues further, and introduced some of the commonly used but less commonly understood terminology used by hospitals, doctors, other healthcare providers, and health insurance plans.

The next chapter addresses a very important issue, you. More specifically, Chapter Five looks at "Taking Care of Your Body."

These are the times that try men's souls.

– Thomas Paine

FIVE

Taking Care of Your Body

The body is a sacred garment. It is your first and
last garment. It is what we enter life with and it
should be treated with honor.

– Martha Graham

*T*he first four chapters of *Living Better* have focused primarily on the world around you, understanding your illness, learning how to have an effective working relationship with your doctors, dealing with hospitals, tests, medications, and financial complications presented by your medical situation. The remainder of the book focuses on various aspects of taking care of yourself, "self-care," in the context of living with life-changing illness.

This chapter covers the key components of taking care of your body, focusing on how you can be proactive in improving your physical situation as much as possible within the limits of your life-changing illness. We call this biological self-care. Subsequent chapters will address the mind-body and mind-body-spirit connection, finding purpose, adjusting your attitude, and nurturing yourself.

This chapter covers the following topics:

- What is Biological Self-Care?

- Nutrition and Illness

    - What Should You Eat?

    - Diet and Osteoporosis

    - Diet and Your Heart

    - Diet and Fiber

    - Sugar and Salt

    - Weight Control

- Exercise and Illness

    - Starting an Exercise Program

    - Deciding How to Exercise

    - Knowing and Managing the Risks of Exercise

- Sleep and Illness

    - The Impact of Not Sleeping Well

    - What If You Can't Sleep?

- Sexuality and Illness

  - Common Misconceptions

  - Rethinking Your View of Sexuality

- Summary

What Is Biological Self-Care?

Biological self-care is accepting responsibility for your health and healing, at least to the extent of doing everything you can to promote healing. However, and we say this loud and clear, *having an illness does not mean that you have done something wrong*! There are many aspects you can't control or don't have much influence over regarding your illness. Nonetheless, there are some very important aspects of your biology—sick or well—where you can have a significant influence on your health.

The self-care we will address in this chapter focuses on eating a nutritious and healthy diet, getting enough exercise, maintaining healthy sleep habits, and dealing with the effects of your illness on your sexuality. These issues were important to your overall health before the onset of your illness. Now that you are dealing with illness, these issues are even more important. You have more at stake and you have the potential to improve your quality of life and help avoid additional chronic problems.

Nutrition and Illness

Someone once said, "You are what you eat." Perhaps this is true. There is no question that your health is in part a product of what you eat. The dietary issues faced by all people are amplified for people living with illness, who have to jump over additional hurdles. You may not be able

> *There is no love sincerer than the love of food.*
>
> – William Shakespeare

to eat certain foods. For example, Carol has difficulty eating fresh fruits and vegetables, foods that would otherwise be very helpful nutritionally and for weight control. Healthy foods may not look good or taste good to you. You may suffer from nausea and queasiness. There is an extra need for creativity in planning and preparing food for chronically ill people.

The things we like to eat are not always what we should eat. One of the challenges of eating right is to reconcile between your *wants* and your *shoulds*. As you focus on this issue, and perhaps put more time and effort into planning for good eating, you are likely to discover healthy foods that you also enjoy.

The discussion of dietary issues in this chapter is based on information provided by Harvard Medical School's Mind/Body Medical Institute. Also, Kristine Napier, M.P.H., R.D. has written an excellent resource for people with chronic illness titled *Power Nutrition for Your Chronic Illness: A Guide to Shopping, Cooking and Eating to Get the Nutrition Edge* (New York: Simon & Schuster MacMillan Co., 1998.) Ms. Napier's nutrition resource includes the basics, special instructions for various diseases, and meal plans that are simple, easy, and delicious. It is hard to find a resource so specific to the needs of people living with chronic illness.

What Should You Eat?

As a rule, Americans do not have healthy eating habits. To help improve the way Americans eat, health experts have developed recommendations for healthy eating. Most of the experts agree on most aspects of a healthy diet. One example is "Dietary Guidelines for Americans" from the U.S.

Department of Agriculture and the U.S. Department of Health and Human Services:

- Eat a variety of foods.

- Maintain a healthy weight.

- Choose a diet low in fat, saturated fat, and cholesterol.

- Choose a diet with plenty of vegetables, fruits, and grain products.

- Use sugars only in moderation.

- Use salt and sodium only in moderation.

- If you drink alcoholic beverages, do so in moderation.

Diet and Osteoporosis

Calcium is important in your diet regardless of your age or your illness. Calcium prevents excessive bone loss, or osteoporosis. The National Institute of Medicine recommends daily calcium intake:

Age 9 to 18	1,300 to 2,500 milligrams (mg)
Age 19 to 50	1,000 to 2,500 mg
Age 51 or more	1,200 to 2,500 mg

Dairy products are excellent sources of calcium. An 8-ounce glass of milk contains about 300 mg of calcium. Yogurts vary from 300 to 400 mg. Most cheeses contain 100 to 200 mg. Leafy green vegetables are another excellent source of calcium.

If you have difficulty getting enough calcium because of your illness, you should consult with your doctor for alternatives. If you have lactose intolerance, for example, you may be able to use tablets or lactose-free milk. In other situations, a calcium supplement may be the solution.

Diet and Your Heart

Whether you are dealing with heart disease or trying to prevent it, eating right is important. Cholesterol levels and fat intake are two interrelated key components of managing your diet to be heart friendly. You should find out your cholesterol levels from your doctor. The tests involve giving the lab a small sample of your blood, usually before you eat breakfast. Most experts recommend a total cholesterol level under 200. LDL, or bad cholesterol, should be below 130, HDL (good cholesterol) should be more than 35 and triglycerides should be below 180. The risk ratio, total cholesterol divided by HDL, should be 4.5 or less, according to most recommendations.

You probably already know to eat a diet with low fat content, but not all fats are created equal. Saturated fats are the main cause of high cholesterol levels. In contrast, unsaturated fats do not raise your cholesterol level. In small amounts they may reduce cholesterol; however, they do contain the same number of calories as saturated fats, so they need to be used in moderation. Olive oil, canola oil, peanut oil, peanut butter, nuts, and avocados are examples of sources of unsaturated fats.

Another type of fat to consider is fish oil, also called Omega-3 fatty acid, whose anti-clotting effect on your blood seems to help protect you from heart disease by reducing your risk of a blocked coronary artery and helping to reduce your level of triglycerides.

Finally, to avoid excessive fat and cholesterol, watch your portions of meat products, keeping them to three-ounce servings.

Diet and Fiber

Adults should consume 20 to 35 grams of fiber per day. Instead, they consume only about 12 grams per day, largely because they eat grain products from which bran has been removed and do not eat enough fruits and vegetables. Here are some recommendations from the American Cancer Society for high-fiber meal planning:

- Use fresh or dried fruits for desserts and snacks.

- Use beans, lentils, and peas.

- Add cooked beans and peas to soups, stews, casseroles, and salads.

- Use nuts and seeds sparingly; they are high in fiber but also high in fat content.

- Eat high-fiber breads and cereals; the first ingredient listed on the package should be a whole grain flour like whole wheat.

- Use grains like buckwheat and brown rice in place of white flour and white rice.

- Leave the skins on potatoes, fruits, and vegetables.

(Brochure titled "Eating Smart," American Cancer Society, 1987.)

Sugar and Salt

Sugar and salt should be a small portion of your diet, yet many Americans consume several times more sugar and salt than their bodies need. Eating fresh foods, rather than processed foods, is one way to get a handle on how much sugar and salt you are consuming. If you have to eat processed foods, read the label. If sodium is one of the first five items listed on the label, the product is probably too high in salt. If you feel like "I can't give up salt, I like the taste," it may help to remember that the taste for salty foods is acquired and can be dis-acquired, too. Lemon, pepper, and other sodium-free spices may help you kick the salt habit.

Weight Control

More than 30 million American adults weigh significantly more than their recommended weight, based on age and height. The potential health benefits of losing weight are too important to pass up, especially for people dealing with other health issues.

You probably know that reducing your weight can help reduce your risk of heart disease, cancer, diabetes, gallbladder disease, and osteoarthritis. Your illness or medications may affect your appetite, your metabolism, and your ability to exercise. These complications make weight control more difficult for people.

We recognize that eating right is easier said than done. We struggle, too. For example, Doug's cholesterol level is above 200. He knows he needs to eat better and exercise more to bring down his total cholesterol and increase his "good" cholesterol. But the immediate enjoyment that an extra slice of beef, a second sandwich, or the "just one" milkshake at the drive-through window can be very alluring, and sometimes irresistible.

In Carol's case, she loves sweets, especially hot fudge sundaes and other chocolate treats. She finds it easier to resist these high-risk treats if there are less harmful snacks around the house, such as crackers, graham crackers and low-fat pudding. She still needs to limit how much of these "extras" she eats, but she is at least able to avoid the more damaging selections.

Remember that the suggestions in this chapter can help you live as well as possible with your illness. But sometimes the cards seem stacked against you! Genetics also play a role. Doug's high cholesterol has a hereditary component, for example. Medications (such as prednisone), your body's ability to tolerate certain foods (affected by chemotherapy or otherwise), and your limitations on exercise (such as being wheelchair bound) play a part in complicating healthy biological self-care.

Psychological factors also bear attention. Sadness, loneliness, depression, anxiety, loss of control and anger at a person, a situation, or your illness can cause lapses from healthy biological self-care. Become aware of how you are feeling and reacting; then try to find healthy ways to care for yourself to avoid unhealthy self-care!

Whatever your eating challenges are, you need to find the best way to reduce the temptations that threaten your long-term health. Making "bad" foods less accessible, such as keeping ice cream out of the house, is one good strategy. Substituting healthy goodies for your favorite foods is another. Whatever it takes, try to find the tactics that work for you. Stick to your plan as best you can. When you lapse, look at why and try to alter your plans to avoid the lapse happening again. All you can do is do the best you can. Talk to your doctor about the best approach for your unique health circumstances.

Exercise and Illness

Healthy Americans need more exercise than they are getting and the same is true for people with chronic illness. With chronic illness, you need to overcome all of the same obstacles to maintaining a regular exercise program as healthy people do. You also must contend with illness-related issues. Within the limits of your specific illness and with your doctor's approval, the benefits of a regular exercise program are too significant for you to pass up.

> The only way to keep your health is to eat what you don't want, drink what you don't like ... and do what you'd rather not.
> – Mark Twain

The American Heart Association says "Be active! It's smart for your heart." (Brochure titled "Just Move!," American Heart Association, 1997.) The Arthritis Foundation says "Exercise is beneficial because it can help ... improve your ability to do daily activities and improve your overall health and fitness by giving you more energy, helping you sleep better and controlling your weight." (Brochure titled "Exercise and Your Arthritis," 1998, Arthritis Foundation.) The Arthritis Foundation offers programs such as water exercise.

The American Heart Association and the Arthritis Foundation are both right. Whether you deal with heart disease, arthritis, or any disease or illness, most of the same principles hold. A regular exercise program can be very beneficial to you. Your specific exercise program needs to be tailored to your unique set of health circumstances, influenced strongly by the type of disease you face. You should consult your physician before you jump right into any exercise program.

The American Heart Association says that regular physical activity offers many benefits that should be attractive to anyone living with illness. Exercise, in conjunction with a proper diet, improves the circulation of blood throughout your body, improves your body's ability to use oxygen, may help you handle stress, bolsters your enthusiasm and optimism, helps you release tension, helps you relax and sleep, and helps you control your weight.

Starting an Exercise Program

Even before getting started, it is important to consider your health and physical capabilities, your interests, facilities, climate conditions, and other factors. Part of this process includes talking to your doctor about exercise before you get started.

Someone once said, "Misery is optional." Those words certainly apply to exercise. Exercise needs to be fun. You need to put an exercise program together that is fun for you. If not, you aren't very likely to stay with the program. Comfort is also important. Make sure you have the seasonally appropriate comfortable clothing and shoes for the activities you choose.

> *Those who think they have not time for bodily exercise will sooner or later have to find time for illness.*
>
> – Edward Stanley,
> 15th Earl of Derby, Circa 1870

When you are getting started, it is important to begin slowly and increase the length and difficulty of your exercising gradually. Most of us have stories we could tell about going "all out" with a new exercise program only to strain a muscle or tendon or ankle, and not be able to continue the activity. Starting gradually and slowly increasing the length of time and the intensity of activity is important for everyone, especially people with chronic illness.

Deciding How to Exercise

Have fun exercising and find exercise activities with repetitive motion using your arms and legs and build endurance.

Activities that increase blood flow to the working muscles for extended periods of time promote "cardiovascular fitness" or endurance. The

American Heart Association suggests activities like walking, hiking, jogging, bicycling, swimming, roller skating and jumping rope. They recommend 30 to 60 minutes of vigorous physical activity three or four times per week. Obviously, your physical limitations need to be taken into consideration. Depending on your circumstances, you may be able to work up to the recommended amount of activity, or perhaps get to 20 minutes. Remember that vigorous activity should not get to the point of you being totally out of breath.

Activities that strengthen your muscles are another component of an effective exercise program. According to Drs. Salt and Season, "Research now shows that you can accomplish the strength and muscular dimension of your self-care and wellness program in as little as 20 to 30 minutes, two to three times a week. Strength can be doubled, fat replaced with muscle." (*Fibromyalgia and The MindBodySpirit Connection: A 7 Step Plan for Living a Healthy Life with Fibromyalgia,* William B. Salt II, M.D. and Edwin H. Season, M.D., Columbus: Parkview, 2000, p. 193). Two books by Ellington Darden, Ph.D., *Living Longer Stronger* (New York: A Perigree Book, 1995) and *Body Defining* (Chicago: Contemporary Books, 1996), and other books by various authors, provide much more specific recommendations for resistance and strength exercise.

Less intense activity is also helpful. Though they lack the dramatic effects of cardiovascular activity, activities like pleasure walking, gardening and dancing are still helpful. These types of activities can be a nice supplement to vigorous activity or a substitute for vigorous activity if your physical condition precludes you from cardiovascular exercise.

For people in wheelchairs who still have some ability to move limbs, look for ideas specific to people with your restriction. Movement is good for everyone. Christopher Reeve has continued exercise with the help of a therapist in order to keep his body as agile and muscular as possible with the hope that he may someday walk again. Group therapies with older adults in nursing homes use large balls to throw back and forth and do a seated version of "head, shoulders, knees, and toes." When exercise is over, their smiles are amazing mood lifters for those helping them as they live within their restrictions.

Knowing and Managing the Risks of Exercise

Considering your physical limitations is a first step, as described above. This includes consulting with your doctor. Once you have determined that you can exercise and have developed a program you are comfortable with, you want to be careful not to do yourself harm.

Warming up is an essential key to managing your risk. Any exercise program should begin with a warm-up period during which breathing rate, circulation, and body temperature increase. Warming up significantly reduces your risk of injury and should last three to five minutes. Your warm up should include stretching the muscles that are going to be called on to do vigorous activity.

After exercising, it is important to cool down for a few minutes. Walk around slowly for a few minutes rather than standing still or lying down. Take time to stretch muscles that feel tight or tense. Let your body slowly readjust to your decreased physical demands.

Keep exercising! Don't stop or compare yourself with other people's activities. Try to accept that your situation is unique to your personality, your interests, and your physical condition. Make sure you are having fun and you are allowing your body to rest between exercise sessions.

Sleep and Illness

You need sleep. Sleep is not an optional activity. The rest that sleep brings your body is essential. You don't have to be living with an illness to need sleep, but if you do live with an illness you are likely to need more sleep and may have difficulty getting the rest you need. Despite stories of some people who can live on three or four hours of sleep, most people need about eight hours of sleep, more or less. Needing more than eight hours of sleep is not something to feel guilty about! Carol needs about 10 hours sleep to keep her from getting run down. At one time, she required 12 hours of sleep per day, nine hours at night plus one or two naps during the day. Extra sleep is just a part of her regimen for living with an illness. She considers rest to be as important as any of her medications.

> *The beginning of health is sleep.*
> – Irish Proverb

Many aspects of sleep remain mysteries which are still not well understood. For example, scientists don't know what triggers the brain and the body to rest rather than remain active or why some people need so much more sleep than others.

Scientists who study sleep do know that there are distinct types and phases of sleep. They know, for example, that your sleep cycles through five stages, starting with Stage 1, a drowsy, relaxed state between waking and sleeping, continuing to Stage 2, the first stage of authentic sleep. In Stage 2, lasting about 30 to 45 minutes, you are still easily awakened. Sleep progresses to Stages 3 and 4, characterized by very slow brain-wave patterns, called delta waves, from which it is difficult to be awakened. In Stages 3 and 4, the heart rate, breathing rate, and other bodily functions drop to their lowest level of the night. Then, after about 45 minutes, you return to Stage 2 for a few minutes, before entering Stage 5, a period of rapid eye movement, or REM, sleep, during which you dream.

If you are having a good night and sleeping soundly, you will progress from Stages 1 to 5 in about 90 minutes and you will go through this cycle four to six times during the night. Sleep tends to get lighter as the night goes on. Toward morning, you tend to wake up briefly, usually falling back to sleep quickly, not remembering that you were awake. (Gregg D. Jacobs, Ph. D., *Say Good Night to Insomnia,* New York: Henry Holt, 1998, pp. 15-17.)

The Impact of Not Sleeping Well

What happens when good sleep doesn't happen? You probably can answer this question from experience. You feel lousy. You are tired, possibly with increased aches, pains, and stiffness. You might feel foggy, not able

> *A ruffled mind makes a restless pillow.*
> – Charlotte Bronte

to think as quickly as you would if you were well rested. You may be in a bad mood, or at least be less tolerant of undesirable and unexpected events. For example, Doug confesses to becoming disproportionately impatient during road construction delays or when other motorists perform stupid driving tricks if he hasn't slept well or enough the night before. He also finds our two dogs' barking, which is usually a little bit irritating, to grate on his nerves like fingernails on a chalkboard if he hasn't slept well the night before.

During deep sleep, the brain and body almost shut down, getting profound rest. Physical energy is renewed. Most of the blood is directed to the muscles, very little to the brain, and the immune system seems to get turned on to combat illness (Jacobs, pp. 17-18.) There is controversy, though, around the issue of how harmful it is to not get enough sleep. Jacobs argues against blaming symptoms on not getting enough sleep, contending that some insomniacs are too quick to assume that bad sleep is the cause of their physical problems. (Jacobs, pp. 78-79.) Bad sleep patterns may or may not contribute to your physical problems.

Jacobs contends that patients sometimes place so much importance on sleep that they feel pressure to fall asleep and even develop a strong fear of insomnia. Doug has a history of mild insomnia, often taking 30 minutes or more to fall asleep, with maybe four or five times a year having an almost sleepless night. At its worst, Doug remembers times when he dreaded nightfall. When it got dark, he became very aware that bedtime was around the corner. As a result, he started to become anxious and fearful of not being able to fall asleep. As he tried to work full-time while dealing with chronic illness, this problem was sometimes amplified because of his perception that he needed to get plenty of sleep and if he didn't, the consequences would include impairing his work performance. When Doug finally overcame the insomnia, it was after he understood self-care essentials, discussed in the next section. Having some technical reading handy as a fallback sleep aid was also helpful.

What If You Can't Sleep?

The National Sleep Foundation offers practical suggestions for improving your sleep. They suggest that a visit with your doctor is the best first step. For people with chronic illness, who probably have a doctor they see frequently, this shouldn't be a problem. Adding sleep problems to your list of questions is a simple step. Your doctor can help determine what underlying problems might contribute to sleep difficulties. Your doctor should also know how your medications might be contributing to sleep problems. The National Sleep Foundation also suggests that you:

1. Avoid caffeine, nicotine, and alcohol in the late afternoon and evening. Caffeine and nicotine can delay sleep, and alcohol may interrupt sleep later in the night.

2. Exercise regularly, but at least three hours before bedtime. Working out too close to bedtime may not give your body a chance to "unwind."

3. If you have trouble sleeping at night, don't nap during the day.

4. Establish a regular, relaxing bedtime routine that will allow you to unwind and send a "signal" to your brain that it's time to sleep. Follow this routine regularly, even on weekends, and build it so that you schedule time for seven to eight hours of sleep.

5. Don't use your bed for anything other than sleep or sex. Your bed should be associated with sleep, not wakefulness.

6. If you can't get to sleep within 30 minutes, get up. Don't stay in bed tossing and turning. Do something relaxing like listening to soothing music or reading. Try to clear your mind but don't use this time to solve your problems.

Your attitude is also important. One fact that may be helpful to remind yourself is that the body's greatest need is for core sleep, the deep sleep during Stages 3 and 4; your body naturally recovers this core sleep, even if you are not aware of it happening.

Thinking positive thoughts can help you sleep better and be less susceptible to insomnia. Here are positive thoughts you can practice if you are concerned or anxious about sleep.

- I am probably getting more hours of sleep than I realize.

- I will be okay as long as I get my core sleep.

- I have lived through sleepless nights before, so I will survive this time.

- After a bad night, I am likely to sleep well the next because my body is focused on catching up on my core sleep.

- If I am having trouble during the day, at least part of it is the result of my negative attitudes toward sleep.

- If I awaken after five or six hours of sleep, I have probably had enough core sleep.

- I will eventually fall asleep during the night as the temperature of my body drops.

- I will eventually feel better later in the day as the temperature of my body rises.

- I can probably improve my sleep gradually by doing things that have worked for other people with similar sleep problems.

Many of the items on this list are things you can try for yourself to see if they help you sleep better. You will probably need to collaborate with your doctor if the simple things don't work. For example, to make sure that your medications aren't causing you sleep problems, you need to talk to your doctor. To pursue medications to help you sleep, you will definitely need to talk to your doctor and work together to determine what medical approach is best for your unique situation.

Some sleep disorders require sleep study, or polysomography, that generally requires an overnight sleep at a specialized sleep study lab. There are several sleep-related breathing disorders, including sleep apnea, whose first symptom is often snoring, that should be evaluated in a sleep lab. Other disorders calling for sleep study include restless legs, periodic movement of limbs, and poor sleep over a long period of time.

Like everything else, your sleep patterns are affected by many factors. If you have sleep difficulty, try to be patient. Some combination of medications, self-care, and other treatments is very likely to help you find more restful sleep.

Sexuality and Illness

"It gives me great pleasure," Winston Churchill said when asked to give an extemporaneous speech on the topic of sex. Sexual intimacy does indeed give most people great pleasure, but people living with illness often have some obstacles to overcome.

Like the other "body" issues in this chapter, sexuality is not exclusively a "body" issue. Your mind and your emotions are integrally involved, but if you are dealing with chronic illness, there are special sexuality issues related to your specific illness and with being chronically ill in general.

You have a normal human need for intimacy, including sexual intimacy. With or without illness, sexuality is often disrupted by physical and emotional problems in your health and in your life; but if you suffer from illness, those problems are often amplified.

Some of these common sexuality issues include:

- You are too tired.

- You are in too much pain.

- Your sexual functions don't function very well.

- Emotional concerns and fears about your illness disrupt your body's sexual chemistry.

- You fear harming yourself.

- Your spouse is less interested for fear of harming you.

(David S. Sobel, M.D., and Robert Ornstein, Ph.D., *The Healthy Mind, Healthy Body Handbook*, DRx: Los Altos, CA, 1998, p. 72.)

Many of these concerns and complications are especially applicable to people coping with heart disease. Author Wayne Sotile, Ph.D., devotes an entire book to *Heart Illness and Intimacy: How Caring Relationships Aid Recovery.* (Baltimore: Johns Hopkins University Press, 1992.) While sexual interaction is just one aspect of intimacy, it is a very important part.

Sometimes healthcare professionals unintentionally convey the feeling that sexual impairment is a minor problem, much less important than high blood pressure for example. Sotile suggests reminding "such a doctor that the only minor sexual problem is one that is happening to someone else." (Sotile, p. 121.) Reality is that intimacy is one of our most basic needs, and marital intimacy is a very important aspect.

Common Misconceptions

The reality of sexual experience is much different from what is portrayed on television and at the movies. Many people see what is portrayed on the screen or in a magazine and compare it to their own reality. They come away with unrealistic expectations and a narrow understanding of what is a healthy sexual relationship. It's probably not a bad idea to challenge many of your expectations and the parameters you place on your sexual relationship with your partner.

There are many misconceptions and misinformation about sexuality. It is very easy to believe what you've heard and seen on television, at the movies, or in music. There are also many common misconceptions about sexual relationships, none of which are helpful. You should consider challenging your thinking if you think that older people can't enjoy sex or that sex is only for beautiful people with beautiful bodies. Other misconceptions are that a man and a woman should always be ready for sex and that sex always means intercourse and orgasm.

Many of these misconceptions are particularly relevant for people who are chronically ill. If you are living with an illness, you may not feel all that great about your body. Disappointment related to sexuality can compound those understandable but unhealthy feelings about your body.

Rethinking Your View of Sexuality

Consider an enlightened approach to sexuality and what sexual intimacy is all about. Drs. Sobel and Ornstein define healthy sex as freely chosen, conscious of consequences, respectful, erotic, playful, a way to be closer, an expression of love and caring. (Sobel and Ornstein, p. 72.)

Although that definition is not directed specifically at people living with an illness, it is still relevant. People with illness have similar problems sexually as other people, often exaggerated by illness. In many cases, perceptions are the culprit, perceptions of what is "normal" and what are illness-related limitations and risks associated with sexual activity.

Sotile's chapter titled "Sex and Heart Illness" suggests that to manage your sex life in a healthy way, there are several key points to remember.

- Every couple copes with differences in sexual drive, response, and preferences. Adjusting to illness simply magnifies these differences.

- It is normal to have periodic difficulties progressing through the sexual response, anywhere from arousal, to plateau and orgasm. Learning to relax without dwelling on past "failures" is an essential part of working through these difficulties.

- Responding sexually is safe for most people, including those with heart disease. Your response may be affected by aging, your medications, and your overall health condition.

- Regardless of your health condition, you can enjoy your sexual relationship more if you apply common sense as you control your behavioral, emotional, and thought patterns surrounding the sexual part of your life.

Your sex life has to do with much more than body parts. Sotile says, "It has to do with the interplay between your own and your partner's most intimate, most vulnerable, and most wonderful layers of that inner sense of self that houses your unique and special gift." (Sotile, p. 138.)

Summary

This chapter has touched on the diverse topics of nutrition, exercise, sleep and sexuality. Much of the content applies to you regardless of your health. If you're dealing with life-changing illness, these issues tend to become more of a challenge to manage in a healthy way.

Acknowledging that your illness changes your life and complicates your biological self-care is realistic and sensible. That doesn't mean that there's nothing you can do to make choices to improve every aspect of your biological self-care. For most people with illness, these issues are challenging but can be managed.

In the next chapter, we will explore the power of your mind-body connection.

Habits are safer than rules; you don't have to keep them. They keep you.

– Frank Crane

SIX

UNDERSTANDING YOUR MIND-
BODY CONNECTION

*The mind, in addition to medicine, has powers
to turn the immune system around.*

– Jonas Salk, M.D.

Your mind and your body are connected. You know that, of course! They are connected by the neck! While that is true, there is much more to the connection than meets the eye. Modern medical science has confirmed with an exploding body of evidence the powerful connection between your mind and your body. Scientists are continuing to develop a better understanding of how the connection works and how it can be used to promote wellness and accelerate healing.

In this chapter we will explore the mind-body connection. The main areas covered in this chapter are listed on the next page.

- Historical Perspective

- The Three-Legged Stool

- Carol's Experience with the Mind-Body Connection

- The Fight-or-Flight Response

- The Relaxation Response

- Why "One"

- Remembered Wellness

- Science of the Mind-Body Connection

- Your Mind-Body Connection

- Warning

- How Change Happens

- Summary

Historical Perspective

The mind-body connection is not new. For example, ancient Greek civilization attributed disease to both physical factors and the mind. The Greeks used the word "Holos," which reflected their understanding that medical disease involved the whole person, not just the diseased part. This is the view still held today in many non-western societies. Our modern term, "holistic medicine," is derived from the same Greek root.

The mind-body connection was taken for granted hundreds and even thousands of years ago. However, philosophers as far back as Plato have suggested a separation between the mind and the body. Viewing the mind and body as separate entities had become the prevailing view by the 16th or 17th century. This view was expressed by French philosopher and mathematician Rene Descartes. In 1637, Descartes suggested that the body did not need the mind to operate.

For the most part, Descartes' suggestion closely matched the prevailing view, especially in the Western world, from his time through most of the 20th century. Disease was considered to be the realm of physicians who used knowledge from the biomedical model only where it could be proven by the logical scientific method. Anything that couldn't be proven scientifically was presumed not to be valid. For all practical purposes, the mind-body connection so commonly talked about today was forgotten.

The rediscovery of the mind-body connection has occurred primarily since about 1975. One of the widely acknowledged pioneers in the rediscovery of the mind-body connection is Harvard Medical School's Dr. Herbert Benson, a cardiologist who wrote *The Relaxation Response*, first published in 1975.

When *The Relaxation Response* was published, the climate was characterized by "expanding reliance on technology, escalating medical costs, and slowly deteriorating doctor-patient relationships." (*The Relaxation Response*, New York: Avon Books, 2000, p. xxiv.) In contrast to this environment, Dr. Benson's book spelled out the connection between the mind and body in a way that could be understood, and eventually accepted by Western scientists, physicians, and patients.

Dr. Benson and his best selling book gained widespread popularity through his appearance with Barbara Walters on ABC's "Good Morning America." Within the last 25 years, between publication of *The Relaxation*

Response and the updated edition quoted above, the medical community as a whole has begun to rediscover the mind-body connection.

Many researchers, including Dr. Benson, have been exploring how this connection works so that it can be "proven" by the scientific method to convince the biomedical community. The Harvard Medical School's Mind/Body Medical Institute, founded in 1988 and honored in 1992 with an endowed Harvard professorship, has been at the forefront of research and application of the mind-body connection.

The Three-Legged Stool

Dr. Benson's model, which you saw in Chapter One, uses a three-legged stool as an analogy for the healthy balance of resources a person can use to obtain health and well being:

- Pharmaceuticals

- Procedures and surgery

- Self-care

Like a three-legged stool, all three legs are essential. Without all three legs, a stool would not be able to stand. The first two legs of Dr. Benson's model, (1) pharmaceuticals and (2) procedures and surgery, fall within the realm of biomedicine, for which implementation requires physicians. However, through the third leg, self-care, each person has the power to use the mind-body connection to enhance his health.

When you have a life-changing illness, just knowing that you have access to some control over your well-being can be very helpful in an otherwise very out of control situation.

To understand how you can use self-care and the mind-body connection to improve your health, having an understanding of the science of the connection is helpful. The Mind/Body Medical Institute's Alice Domar, Ph.D., describes mind-body medicine as "any method in which the mind is mobilized in the treatment of a physical disorder." (*Self-Nurture: Learning to Care for Yourself as Effectively as You Care for Everyone Else,* New York: Viking Penguin, 2000, p. 5.)

Domar describes five areas of mind-body techniques:

- Relaxation

- Cognitive restructuring (changing negative thought patterns)

- Emotional expression

- Skills for communication and coping

- Spiritual practices

(Domar, p. 5.)

Throughout the remaining chapters you will be learning how to implement these techniques in your life. Later in this chapter we will describe the science that is behind the mind-body connection in both everyday and scientific terms. First we will explore a real-life example of the mind-body connection.

Carol's Experience with the Mind-Body Connection

Carol realized the profound effect of the mind over her body during one of her many hospital stays. At the time, two specialists were caring for two different problems. One of the doctors was the cardiologist who had started Carol on an experimental medication for a heart rhythm disturbance. The other was a gastroenterologist called in for an unrelated procedure, who was filling in for her trusted specialist.

One day she recalls that blood tests had been ordered to be done every half-hour for a research regimen for an experimental medication she was trying. This presented a major problem; under the best of circumstances Carol's veins do not tolerate drawing of blood or insertion of intravenous (IV) needles. This same day a doctor who was not familiar with her scheduled Carol for an esophageal procedure. The esophageal procedure required an additional IV line for injection of a sedative.

As Carol was repeatedly poked unsuccessfully for an IV, she was also being poked for the regularly scheduled blood work. Because the doctors, nurses, and lab technicians were unable to find a vein, they *eventually* injected the sedation in her hip. The doctor then suggested she relax for a half-hour before they do the procedure.

Relax? Carol tried her best but her body was not easily taken over when it was threatened by an esophageal procedure and more blood draws. The esophageal procedure was aborted because she was not sedated, even though she had received enough drugs to "snocker an elephant."

As soon as Carol was returned to her room she was accosted by another appeal for blood. This time, they were able to put in an IV lead so that Carol would not require any more needle sticks. As the lab technician left the room, Carol began to hear a buzz in her head...Good night...The medicine could now work...her fears of further assaults on her veins had abated and her body could finally relax!

The Fight-or-Flight Response

We will start to explain the science of the mind-body connection by focusing on three processes you may already recognize. These three processes are:

- The fight-or-flight response

- The relaxation response

- Remembered wellness

> *You have the power to heal and this comes from you. Everyone—people, patients, and doctors—tends to underestimate this power and potential.*
> – William B. Salt II. M.D. and Edwin H. Season, M.D.

First we will focus on the fight-or-flight response, which was at work in Carol in the previous example. Imagine the following situation. A mother sees her child trapped under her car in the driveway. She runs with all her might, grabs the car bumper with her hands and lifts the car. Using her foot, as both her hands are holding the car, she moves her child away from the tire, saving his life.

You might be asking, "How can she do that?" Unless you are very unusual, you couldn't go to your car in the garage right now and accomplish that feat. You almost certainly wouldn't even try. But stories such as this happen from time to time. You read about these stories in your local newspaper. These events happen so you probably assume there must be a reason. There is.

The reason these seemingly impossible events occur is a physical reaction to perceived danger. This physical reaction is called the fight-or-flight response. Around 1900, Harvard Medical School's Dr. Walter B. Cannon discovered this mechanism in all human bodies.

You have experienced the fight-or-flight response, just as the young mother above experienced it, even if you haven't had such a dramatic experience. Your body is able to produce this same kind of physiological response that would allow you to be able to lift your car!

This same response enabled your caveman relatives to carry their children to safety from saber-tooth tigers. Even today, in extreme situations such as saving a child's life, this fight-or-flight response is a healthy response.

These physiological changes did an excellent job at what they were created to do for our prehistoric relatives. The problem today is that even now our human bodies continue to be "hard-wired" to respond to stressful situations, as observed in the mind, with a fight-or-flight response. However, modern human bodies still react to their stressful thoughts as if saber-tooth tigers are a constant threat. Human bodies are not designed to stay on continuous alert to maintain these physiological responses on a frequent or ongoing basis.

With each new stressful event, your body becomes more and more alert and aroused, which in turn can cause many physical responses in your body. Producing these fight-or-flight responses all day long (as often as 50 times each day) causes wear and tear on 21st century humans. These physical responses are harmful over a long period of time and can actually make your body sick and more susceptible to illness.

Responding daily and repeatedly to stress works against the health of your body because each new encounter during the day increases the arousal level without returning the body to the pre-stress level. Stated another way, the baseline of your arousal reactions steadily moves upward. If you can learn how to encourage your body back into a healthy pre-stress state after a stressful event has provoked the fight-or-flight response, then you can reduce the damage caused by your body's ongoing physical response to stress.

Back in the era when cavemen fought off saber-tooth tigers, this response was necessary for survival. Today, it decreases your body's capability to survive. Today, this bodily response is generally not very useful. People with life-changing illness, whose bodies are already compromised, do not need the effects of needless fight-or-flight responses.

The following section on the relaxation response gives you a method to lower your arousal from fight-or-flight and to regain your pre-stress state.

The Relaxation Response

More than 60 years after Dr. Cannon discovered the fight-or-flight response at Harvard, Harvard's Dr. Herbert Benson discovered its antidote in the same room. Benson was looking for an effective method for patients to lower blood pressure which would have fewer side effects than the available medications. Benson named this behavioral antidote to fight-or-flight, "the relaxation response."

> *Tension is who you think you should be.*
>
> *Relaxation is who you are.*
>
> – Tai Chi Expression

The relaxation response is the opposite reaction within your body to the fight-or-flight response. It has many immediate biological responses within your body. Dr. Benson found that the relaxation response resulted in lower blood pressure by provoking a state of bodily calm. In turn, the response then affects your body by not only lowering blood pressure, but also by lower heart, breathing, and metabolic rates. Through these changes, the relaxation response thus can quiet the effects of the fight-or-flight response.

The relaxation response was the initial component of self-care that Dr. Benson incorporated into his practice of medicine. This technique is now used in a variety of medical symptom reduction groups at the Mind/Body Medical Institute. These groups include pain reduction, menopause, cancer, AIDS, infertility, cardiac rehabilitation, and insomnia. The relaxation response has become the cornerstone for helping you to help your body remember how to relax.

With chronic illness, you need a safe haven. You need to find a place of calm, a place of control when your health seems out of control. The relaxation response can be a way for you to find that essential place of calm. The technique is very simple to explain and to do. There are generally no harmful side effects. The challenge is to change your life and to do the exercise on a consistent basis! Changing is very difficult. We will discuss making changes in your life and how you can to do it later in this chapter.

As we discussed earlier, your body has as many as 50 fight-or-flight responses every day. You will also find that the responses from either the fight-or-flight reaction or the relaxation response continue to carry over throughout your day. Common sense tells you it is to your benefit to regularly evoke the relaxation response.

There are many ways to trigger or evoke the relaxation response, including prayer, exercise, yoga, and breathing exercises. Dr. Benson says that the common ingredient of all these techniques is a two-step process.

Step 1. Repeat and focus on a word, sound, prayer, phrase, or muscular activity.

Step 2. Passively disregard everyday thoughts that come to mind, and return to your repetition.

(Benson, *The Relaxation Response*, 2000, p. 134.)

In Step 1, examples of words you can repeat and focus on include *peace, calm, relax, Our Father who art in heaven, The Lord is my shepherd, Hail Mary,* and *Shalom.* For some people, staying still is very difficult. Depending on what is best for you, you may also take a walk or do yoga, focusing on your breath and the repetitive motion of the activity. Taking a walk at a steady pace in which you focus on each step you take can be an excellent way to evoke the relaxation response if you find it too difficult to sit still and concentrate.

Step 2 is to passively disregard thoughts. This is very challenging for today's busy minds. Americans have become very adept at multitasking. Doug frequently reads the newspaper, eats breakfast, feeds or lets in or lets out the dogs, listens to the radio, and checks e-mail, all at the same time. The wise Bible passage "be still and know that I am God" is seldom obeyed today. Your mind is often cluttered with all kinds of thoughts, all the time. You may be consciously aware of some thoughts but unconscious of others. There can be a silent running dialogue within you that sometimes includes negative attitudes and stress-producing ideas. As you begin to try the relaxation response, be aware that everyone has intrusive thoughts. As you practice the technique, you will get better at shutting these thoughts down, but don't be hard on yourself now. Just passively acknowledge the thought and then disregard the thought and let it go.

The environment for eliciting the response is also important. Try to find a quiet place that can be free from interruptions for 20 minutes. While this may seem impossible, it can be made possible with some forethought. You may want to let your phone calls be answered by voice mail, put the pets outside, and find a time when other members of your household are occupied. Other members of your household may need to learn to respect your need for uninterrupted time.

Many people do not believe they can find this much time for themselves. If you are one of these people, then try to begin to change this thinking pattern. Everyone needs and deserves this small amount of time as a minimum for personal self-care. Remember that your body is hard-wired for both the fight-or-flight response and the relaxation response. Both of these are your birthright. To use the relaxation response effectively, you must exercise this birthright by practicing how to evoke it on a regular basis. Even though you have not been aware of it, you have been practicing the fight-or-flight response for years; now it is time to practice the relaxation response.

Here is the relaxation response technique, with more detail, as described by Dr. Benson. (*Timeless Healing: The Power and Biology of Belief*, Scribner: New York, 1996, p. 136.) (Note that our comments are indicated by parentheses.)

- **Focus on a word or phrase.** Pick a focus word or short phrase that's firmly rooted in your belief system.

- **Sit comfortably.** Sit quietly in a comfortable position. (Most often this is sitting up straight in a chair with arms comfortably relaxed in your lap. Try to reserve the same place and time each day to help the response become a habit.)

- **Close your eyes.** (Some people are not comfortable with closing their eyes. If you have been traumatized for some reason, closing your eyes may feel unsafe. If this is so for you, just leave your eyes open.)

- **Relax your muscles.** (Focus on various muscle groups, one by one. For example, focus on relaxing your neck and shoulder muscles, then your arms, then your wrists, and then your hands and fingers.)

- **Breathe slowly and naturally.** As you breathe slowly and naturally, repeat your focus word, phrase or prayer, silently to yourself as you exhale. (Notice where in your chest your breath comes. It should be deep in your abdomen and your belly button should be rising and falling, your shoulders and upper chest barely moving. This is called diaphragmatic breathing.)

- **Have a passive attitude.** Assume a passive attitude. It is quite normal for your mind to wander. Don't worry about how well you're doing. When these or other thoughts come to mind, simply say to yourself, "Oh well," and gently return to the repetition.

- **Continue for 10 to 20 minutes.** (You may need to start with a shorter time. Set an alarm that will not jolt you from relaxation, but that will alert you that your time has ended.)

- **Return slowly.** Do not stand immediately. Continue sitting quietly for a minute or so, allowing other thoughts to return. Then open your eyes if they were closed and sit for another minute before rising. (The technique does work and often your blood pressure has lowered, so be cautious when you stand because you may be light-headed momentarily.)

- **Practice this technique once or twice daily.** (You may want to keep some notes on how you feel before and after practicing the relaxation response, especially during the first two weeks.)

The Mind/Body Medical Institute has an alternative it calls "minis" for people who have trouble finding 20 minutes to evoke the relaxation response. A mini is a shortened version that takes one to two minutes and yet it can have an impact on those 50 or more daily fight-or-flight moments. Minis help decrease your fight-or-flight responses. Mini relaxation exercises are focused breathing techniques that help reduce anxiety and tension immediately. Minis can be done with your eyes open or closed—although open eyes are recommended while driving! They can be done with the people around you being totally unaware you are doing them. Try to make a habit of doing minis throughout the day. Every time you do a mini when you meet a stressful situation, you help counteract the stress reaction in your body. Just as the stress response compounds with multiple events, the relaxation response can become stronger the more it is called into action.

Here are three versions of minis taught at the Mind/Body Medical Institute:

- **Count down.** Count very slowly to yourself from ten down to zero, one number with each deep diaphragmatic breath. When you get to zero, see how you are feeling. If you are still stressed out, repeat the exercise.

- **Count up.** As you inhale, count very slowly up to four; as you exhale, count slowly back down to one. Thus, as you inhale, you say to yourself "one, two, three, four." Then as you exhale, you say to yourself "four, three, two, one." Do this exercise several times.

- **Pause.** After each breath, pause for a few seconds. After you exhale, pause again for a few seconds. Do this exercise for several breaths.

The Mind/Body Medical Institute suggests that there are many good times to do a mini.

- When you are stuck in traffic

- Waiting on hold during an important phone call

- When you are waiting in your doctor's office

- When someone says something that bothers you

- When sitting at a red light

- While waiting for a phone call

- When you are in the dentist's chair

- When you are overwhelmed by what you need to accomplish

- When you are waiting in line

- While you are experiencing pain

We have included the following list of relaxation response techniques. You can use these exercises to elicit the relaxation response beyond the basic approach already described. These techniques fit different individual tastes and needs, so you can find the most comfortable program for you.

- **Breath awareness and diaphragmatic breathing.** With this exercise you learn to breathe so that the body efficiently gives itself adequate air. This is done by breathing from deep in your abdomen, allowing your abdomen to rise and fall with each breath. This is sometimes called belly breathing. Often you breathe short, shallow breaths with only your shoulders rising and falling. Try clenching your fists, now notice how you are breathing (most likely if you are breathing at all the breath is not in the abdomen and diaphragm). Now relax your fist and breathe deeply. How do you feel different? The key is to concentrate on the in and out breaths, allowing other thoughts to passively drift from your consciousness. By putting your hands across your abdomen, you can observe whether the abdomen or the upper chest and shoulders are moving up and down. Most of the movement should be in your abdomen to provide room for air to move into the lungs.

- **Body awareness and body scan.** This exercise helps you become aware of tense areas in your body. First, begin with breathing as discussed above; then, close your eyes (if you are comfortable with doing so) and become aware of the sounds, smells, and sensations within the room by thinking "I am aware of the sounds outside, the sounds in the house, in this room…." Pause between thoughts to allow time for observation. Next draw your thoughts inward and become aware of your inner self. For example, is your nose itching or your stomach growling? Go back and forth between inner and outer worlds for a few minutes in order to separate the two worlds. Then scan your body, one part at a time, becoming aware of how it feels. Begin with your head and end with your toes, consciously becoming aware of tension and relaxation. End with several healthy breaths by breathing deep in your abdomen so that your stomach rises and falls and so that your shoulders stay almost still.

- **Progressive muscle relaxation.** With this technique each muscle group is tensed and then relaxed so that you can sense the difference between a state of tenseness and relaxation. Closing your eyes along with the breathing technique aids in focusing and relaxing you.

When you begin to tense and relax each muscle group, give yourself some word cues in your mind such as letting go, smoothing out the muscle, or calming the muscles. This exercise may be shortened to use in your work office or in a visit to your physician's office by simply focusing on several muscle groups, such as the forehead (wrinkling), the hands (clenching), and the back (arching).

- **Prayer and other ways to practice meditation.** Many people use various forms of meditation, which produce a state of relaxation using their individual faith practices. Ron DelBene describes the breath prayer or Jesus Prayer, which Christians have used since the very beginnings of their faith history. (*The Hunger of the Heart Workbook*, Nashville: Upper Room, 1995, pp. 147-148.) DelBene suggests the following routine:

    - Focus on the breath, as previously described in "Breath Awareness and Diaphragmatic Breathing."

    - Next recall a calming passage from the Bible.

    - As you continue with your eyes closed, imagine that God calls your name and asks you, "What do you need?" or "What do you want that will make you feel most whole?"

    - In your mind, answer God directly with what comes from your heart in a simple, short answer.

    - Next choose your favorite name or image of God.

    - Put your answers (to the questions "What do you need?" and "What do you want that will make you feel most whole?") together with your one or two-word image of God. You can put together a prayer/meditation that is similar to the following examples: "Good Shepherd, give me rest," "Yahweh, I need shalom," or "Jesus, take away my pain."

- As you breathe in and out slowly and rhythmically, focus on the words you have chosen.

These examples are based on Christianity and Judaism. Other faiths use variations on this relaxation technique. We encourage you to use a variation that is most comfortable and consistent with your belief system.

- **Guided imagery.** This is a gentle but powerful technique, described by Belleruth Naparstek as "directed daydreaming," that focuses and directs the imagination. Imagery involves all of the senses, and almost anyone can do this. People can invent their own imagery, or they can listen to imagery that's been created for them (see Web page www.healthjourneys.com for resources). To begin, as in the other techniques, focus on the breath and becoming relaxed. Use your sensory images. At first with help from a tape, walk yourself through a story about a safe place you create using mental images and sensations that give you a sense of calm. Music that is soothing is also helpful for this and other techniques. For this method we recommend you begin with a guided imagery tape recording produced by a knowledgeable source. Gradually, you may wish to find your own words for description, possibly even making your own tape.

- **Yoga stretching.** Yoga stretching is based on 3,000 year-old Indian philosophy. Yoga combines centering and slow focused breathing with gentle physical postures and movements. Yoga stretching is used with the patients who come to the Mind/Body Medical

Institute. The exercises are done while sitting, standing, or lying on the floor and can be modified for those who have chronic conditions that may make a certain position or movement difficult. Yoga can be very beneficial and can be practiced without altering your religious beliefs or accepting a new religion or philosophy. If yoga is new to you, check out a beginner video or try a class at a recreation center, school, church, or wellness center in your community.

- **Mindfulness.** The concept of mindfulness is based on Tibetan Buddhism and is both a philosophy and a relaxation practice. Simply stated, mindfulness is about being present in the moment. Mindfulness is the opposite of worrying about past or present or having specific expectations for your life, or taking life for granted. It is being aware of what is happening with all of your senses *moment by moment.* Try opening a candy bar mindfully. Think about how the package looks, how the candy bar smells, and how it feels in your hand, for example. With this practice you can rediscover pleasure in the smallest of activities. It allows you to focus and relax your mind, which in turn changes your body physiologically.

- **Autogenic training.** This approach is a systematic program that will teach your body and mind to respond quickly and effectively to your verbal commands to relax and return to a balanced, normal state. With concentration you scan your body repeating phrases such as my right arm is heavy… my right arm is warm… my right arm is heavy and warm… This can be used in conjunction with biofeedback. Biofeedback uses instruments to detect and amplify specific physical states in your body that you usually don't notice and to help bring them voluntary control. We would not recommend you start by learning about relaxation with this method, because this method entails more steps.

Several books describe these techniques in detail, including *The Wellness Book: The Comprehensive Guide to Maintaining Health and Treating Stress-Related Illness* (Herbert Benson, Eileen M. Stuart, Fireside, 1993), *The Relaxation and Stress Reduction Workbook* (Martha Davis, Elizabeth Eshelman and Matthew McKay, New York: New Harbinger, 1995), and *Healing Mind, Healthy Woman* (Alice Domar, Ph.D., and Henry Dreher, New York: Delta/Dell, 1996.) In addition to in-depth descriptions of how to do these methods, the following organizations and their Web sites recommend resources on tape that will help coach you through learning the process.

- **Harvard Medical School's Mind/Body Medical Institute.** Attn: Tapes, 110 Francis Street, Suite 1A, Boston, MA 02215, (617) 632-9530. The Institute's tapes also include information on the basics of relaxation, progressive muscle relaxation, and examples of guided imagery. In addition to these techniques, tapes are available using practices such as yoga for relaxation. Their Web address is www.mindbody.harvard.edu/orderinga.htm#top.

- **Health Journeys.** Image Paths, Inc., P.O. Box 5714, Cleveland, OH 44101. Resources include a book about using guided imagery, *Staying Well With Guided Imagery: How to Harness the Power of Your Imagination for Health and Healing* by Belleruth Naparstek (Warner Books: New York, 1994) that is intended for people with illness, who are seeking healing and health. Naparstek also has a large selection of excellent tapes available that can be found in bookstores. At the Web site, www.healthjourneys.com, you can sample audio files from the tapes. Naparstek's tapes use the type of relaxation we described as guided imagery. Her guided imagery tapes use descriptive words and music to guide the listener on an inner journey to health wellness.

- **New Harbinger Publications, Inc..** 5674 Shattuck Avenue, Oakland, CA 94609, (800) 748-6273. New Harbinger offers self-help, psychology and health publications and tapes, as well as online exercises. Their Web address is www.newharbinger.com.

Why "One"

You may have heard some people inaccurately describe the relaxation response as a religious ritual. Dr. Benson believes that this misunderstanding results from the common use of "one" as the point of focus, suggesting to some a link to Eastern religion. You may not have heard the rest of the story.

Focusing on "one" is often suggested to people using the relaxation response because researchers found this to work best with their research subjects. Dr. Benson had initially asked the research subjects to count ten breaths. Unfortunately, the subjects could not keep track of counting to ten. The research subjects, Harvard students, lost count! Dr. Benson then suggested they just focus on the number one.

From now on, if people tell you that the relaxation response is a spiritual ritual, you can tell them it is not. Harvard students just can't count! It is true that evoking the relaxation response can include a spiritual term that you are comfortable with. Many people do this, with great success in the context of many spiritual traditions. Dr. Benson has "discovered" something that religious traditions of the world have known was good for us for thousands of years!

Remembered Wellness

Now that we have covered the fight-or-flight response and the relaxation response, we will turn to the third component of mind/body medicine, remembered wellness.

In *Timeless Healing: The Power and Biology of Belief,* Dr. Benson describes his life-long fascination with the connection between the mind and body and his theories on how it works. As Dr. Benson has continued to study the relaxation response, he has made some further realizations about the power of self-care and how integrating self-care in one's lifestyle can be beneficial to one's health and well-being.

Along with learning how to evoke this calming relaxation response, Dr. Benson realized that there is what he describes as "a remembered wellness" inside each of us that has a very potent healing effect. This remembered wellness includes the placebo effect. The "Microsoft Encarta Online Encyclopedia" defines *placebo* as follows:

> An inert substance used instead of an active drug to avoid bias in testing new drugs. In a blind test, patients do not know if they have been given the active drug or the placebo; in a double-blind test, physicians observing the results also do not know. Placebos are sometimes given to patients, often inducing an improvement, at least temporarily, of the patient's condition.

Dr. Benson's research sought to show the difference between the relaxation response and the placebo effect. As he went about this research, he discovered a state he named "remembered wellness." The placebo effect is just one aspect of remembered wellness.

Dr. Benson believes that the placebo effect is contained in our hard-wired belief and memory of wellness deep within each of us. He describes that during his research:

> …I began to realize the power of self-care, the healthy things that individuals can do for themselves. More and more, I became convinced that our bodies are wired to benefit from exercising not only our muscles but also our rich inner, human core—our beliefs, values, thoughts and feelings. I was reluctant to explore these factors because philosophers and scientists have, through the ages, considered them intangible and unmeasurable, making any study of them "unscientific." But I wanted to try because again and again, my patients' progress and recoveries often seemed to hinge upon their spirit and will to live. And I could not shake the sense I had that the human mind—and the beliefs we so often associate with the human soul—had physical manifestations. (*Timeless Healing*, p. 17.)

Dr. Benson and many physicians, scientists, and psychologists are gaining a new level of understanding of how you can affect your own health through self-care that will create physiological changes within your body. Throughout the rest of this book we will describe how you can change your thoughts, feelings and actions and thus change the state of your body.

Science of the Mind-Body Connection

For those of you interested in the science behind this concept and how the mind and body work together, we are including the following science lesson, which we hope you find as fascinating as we do. Learning how to evoke the desired responses can produce positive results in every area of your life, including the health of your physical body!

The fight-or-flight response begins with a *perception* of a threat by the brain's cortex. This perception may come from an outward sensing and/or an inward belief to which your brain reacts. The reaction may be valid or invalid. Nevertheless, the brain's perception is of threat and the brain reacts as if there is a reason for fear and intense stress.

Two tiny masses inside your head react to the perceived threat. One is the hypothalamus, which is inside your brain. The second is the pituitary gland, underneath and almost surrounded by the brain. The pituitary is often called the master gland of the endocrine system.

The hypothalamus and pituitary react, provoking a multitude of reactions within the body that essentially prepared the caveman's body to run for its life when called upon. Because this response allowed Mr. Caveman to live so that he could pass on this mechanism, modern humans have a brain and body elaborately set up for the fight-or-flight response. This complex response goes something like this:

- **Recognition of threat.** The brain recognizes a threat, through sensory inputs and beliefs already learned, and communicates the threat to the hypothalamus. As a result, the hypothalamus communicates the threat to the pituitary gland which sends the body a hormone called ACTH.

- **Physical responses.** These actions by the brain, hypothalamus, and the pituitary gland have certain short-term and long-term effects on physical responses of the body. These responses all form a perception in the brain of fear or other stressful emotion such as anger. For example, cortisol, one of the hormones which increases in this response, has widespread and dramatic somatic (body) effects.

- **Sodium retention.** Sodium is retained and vascular reactivity is enhanced, which in turn causes increased blood pressure.

- **Blood clotting.** Coagulability of blood is increased, which increases the risk of a blood clot.

- **Increased lipids.** Lipids increase as a result of a process, which stimulates the mobilization of adipose tissue fat.

- **Increased blood sugar.** Increased blood sugar and decreased immune system response are also the result of the increase in cortisol.

Look at the following table from the Mind/Body Medical Institute showing how fear affects the entire body.

An Event Happens		
The Brain Perceives a Threat		
The Brain Tells the Pituitary and the Hypothalamus to Produce Important Secretions for the Body to Respond to the Event		
The Secretions Affect the Following		
Central Nervous System	Somatic Motor System	Autonomic Nervous System
Perception narrowed	Tension in muscles	Increase in:
Memory coarse and imprecise	Ready for action	• Heart rate
Learning blocked	Jaws clenched	• Blood pressure
Conditioning defense		• Oxygen needs
Tendency to regress or preserve		• Breathing rate
Expectancies are negative		• Blood sugar
Tone is flee or destroy		Adrenalin flows
		Digestive track shuts down
		Blood goes to large muscles, vessels in hands and face constrict

The reality of this science is simple: *your mind can and does affect your body*. That is good news for people with chronic illness. You have at your fingertips, within yourself, the tools to improve your life and your health and well-being. Now you need to learn how to use these tools to benefit yourself rather than hurting your body. (If you are already feeling guilty that maybe you could have changed your health, you may want to move forward to the section titled "Warning" later in this chapter.)

Your Mind-Body Connection

Earlier in this chapter we used the rare example of the mother who was able to pick up a car to save her child. There are other more common ways to be aware of this elaborate physical connection between mind and body. On a smaller scale you may have experienced the mind-body connection yourself in some common situations. You may have

- Awakened with "butterflies" in your stomach the day of a test.

- Been aware of the funny feeling that you feel when you "fall in love."

- Had stomach cramps before an important athletic event.

- Noticed sweaty palms before speaking to a group.

- Experienced diarrhea after a traumatic event.

- Had your heart "ache" when a loved one died.

All of these are examples of the thoughts in your mind and your body responding to the thoughts. You don't just perceive an event in your mind. You also perceive it in your body. Even more amazing is that often when you can close your eyes and think about the event, you have the same bodily reactions days, months, or even years later. Your body reacts to visualized memory in your brain with chemical reactions as if the event were actually occurring in the present. Thus, you can remember the past event with sensations similar to those you experienced when the original event happened.

Think of some of the more exciting, embarrassing, or otherwise emotional events you may have experienced. Ask yourself some questions.

- Can you smell your lover's perfume?

- Do you get goose bumps on your arms when you think of a past event?

- Do you feel cramps or a tightening in your stomach at the thought of a final exam?

- Can you taste the lemon in Grandma's fresh lemonade or smell her homemade pie?

A different and more profound example of the mind-body connection is Post-Traumatic Stress Disorder. PTSD is a psychological description of the reaction of a person who has been through a traumatic event. The body of a person with PTSD reacts as if the event is happening in the present. You may be familiar with one example of this from stories of combat veterans who hear a car backfire and dive for cover behind the nearest parked car. Are they crazy? Most certainly not! Their bodies are connecting with the self-preservation part of the brain, which does not have the luxury to take time to consciously sort out whether the sound was heard today or just remembered. The sound seems like a gun in the battlefield, so the body and mind think they "know" how to react without hesitation.

When the human body learned this reaction in the battlefield, it was a healthy reaction. But in normal modern daily life it is generally not convenient or productive to dive for the nearest parked car. In the example, the automatic, nonthinking response is what would be called a dysfunctional mind-body reaction. Although most people do not have such dramatic mind-body reactions, they have reactions similar to the ones described just prior to the discussion of PTSD. These reactions are not particularly helpful for you today, either.

The above examples illustrate situations in which a thought produces a reaction in your body. Your mind and its thoughts can affect your illness and health. Similarly, disease or illness in the body can affect the mind. For example, think about the last time you or a friend had a "miserable" cold. Is the cold miserable in your body or are you feeling miserable in your mind?

How does a "miserable" cold feel to your body?

- Perhaps your nose feels all stopped up.

- Your throat is sore.

- Your muscles may ache.

- You may have sensations of thirst or a queasy stomach.

How does a "miserable" cold feel to your mind?

- You need to be left alone.

- You want someone to hold you.

- You feel out of control and powerless.

- You feel guilty that you can't accomplish something you have promised.

We all have at one time or another had a cold and felt some or all of these symptoms. Consider that those body sensations and feelings in the head are in response to a simple three-day cold. Imagine the extent of interaction between your longer-term illness, your emotions and every aspect of your body and mind.

How your body and your mind react can seem very involuntary and far from your conscious control. Nonetheless, you can take control of your self-care. You can exercise more control than you might imagine with important aspects of the mind-body connection.

Warning

We need to issue one warning before we continue. The potential of the mind-body connection and the relaxation response is a reason to rejoice. However, the possibility of receiving benefits is not a reason to lay a guilt trip on yourself or your loved ones for not "doing it well enough" to get well or, worst yet, for causing your illness in the first place.

We believe that Dr. Joan Borysenko makes this point effectively in saying:

> Take a look at the lives of saints if you are convinced that thinking right will have you live forever. They all die. For the most part, saints die of just what everybody else does. They die from cancer and heart disease.
>
> (Joan Borysenko, Ph.D., "Spirituality & Healing," recorded during 8th International Psychology of Health, Immunity, and Disease Conference, Sounds True Recordings, © 1996.)

Remember Dr. Herbert Benson's analogy, the three-legged stool of healing mentioned in Chapter One and earlier in this chapter: (1) pharmaceuticals, (2) procedures and surgery, and (3) self-care. Advocating self-care and recognizing the power of your mind-body connection doesn't imply that you abandon other tools available to you and your team of healthcare professionals. You know that medications and medical/surgical interventions, such as surgery and other procedures, are helpful to many people, including you. Just as controlling the mind-body connection through skillful self-care doesn't work perfectly, neither do pharmaceuticals and procedures and surgery work perfectly.

Scientists and practitioners are constantly discovering improvements in all three legs of the healing stool. Also the three legs are not independent of one another. They must work together. Someone with a cancerous tumor must use pharmaceuticals, in the form of chemotherapy, surgery to remove a tumor, and procedures such as radiation to conquer the cancerous disease. When you invoke the mind-body connection with self-care, you still want to use the other two legs of the stool.

In addition, there are many other factors, such as environment and genetics, which you can't necessarily choose. Examples include your family's history of heart disease or cancer or having lived in an environment with extreme air pollution. We urge you not to let yourself feel like a failure if you do not get well. Thinking *wouldda, couldda, shouldda* (would have, could have, should have) thoughts do nothing to help you feel better or live better or longer. So please don't beat up yourself or your loved ones because self-care has not cured your illness. Pat yourself on the back for what you are doing right today.

How Change Happens

Someone said, "If you keep doing what you already did, then you will get what you already got." Another way to express the same sentiment about change is, "Insanity is doing the same thing over and over again and expecting the result to be different." A Greek philosopher said, "You may have habits that weaken you. The secret of change is to focus all your energy, not on fighting the old, but on building the new."

No one ever said changing a life-long, habitual way of doing something was easy! You would probably agree that as long as you keep doing the same behaviors and having the same thoughts, you are going to continue to have the feelings. Nothing much will be any different. Accepting that you can change, learning how to change, and empowering yourself are essential concepts to implement many of the ideas in this book.

"Even when we're aware of the benefits of change, there's often a gap between thinking about it and doing it. Understanding the nature of change helps bridge that gap, increasing the odds that your new efforts will be successful and lasting." (*The Healthy Mind, Healthy Body Handbook*, by David S. Sobel, M.D., and Robert Ornstein, Ph.D., Los Altos, CA: DRx, 1996, p. 17.) This section will help you bridge the gap between knowing about and desiring healthful change, and in doing it.

Sometimes change happens without much effort on your part. You change the style of your clothing, you change your hairstyle, you learn a new card game, or you learn how to drive a car. However, putting the ideas of this book into practice is about learning new knowledge and changing old patterns. Drs. Sobel and Ornstein (Sobel and Ornstein, pp.

18-19) describe three types of change: "pleasurable change," "breakthrough change," and "step-by-step change," as described next:

- **Pleasurable change.** This is the easiest type of change. Sobel and Ornstein suggest that you pick the easiest and most fun things to change first. Improving your environment with music that picks you up or calms you down, taking a siesta, taking time to visit a favorite park, or playing with a pet are easier changes because they make you feel good. These changes can give you a new sense of control over your life. This new confidence, that you have some control, can encourage you to make more difficult changes.

- **Breakthrough change.** As we discussed in Chapter One, the Chinese word for crisis combines the symbols for danger and opportunity. You have probably seen someone diagnosed with heart disease or cancer suddenly lose the weight they have wanted to lose for many years or finally stopped smoking "for good" even though they have unsuccessfully tried many times. These people are using their health crisis as the opportunity and reason to make important changes in their lives.

- **Step-by-step change.** Authors Prochaska, Diclemente, and Norcross labeled this method of change. These authors report on their findings from years of research that they have done concerning how people change habits. In their book *Changing for Good: A Revolutionary Six-Stage Program for Overcoming Bad Habits and Moving Your Life Positively Forward*, they outline the process of change and how to make those changes. (James O. Prochaska, Ph.D., John C. Norcross, Ph.D., and Carlo C. Diclemente, Ph.D., New York: Avon Books, 1994, pp. 38-46.)

According to Drs. Prochaska, Diclemente, and Norcross, there are six levels of change that each person goes through in making a "step-by-step" change. Often a person will try the wrong processes to facilitate change. If the person making the change or his or her family and other support people do not realize where in the change process that person is, change may be thwarted and often the person fails at the attempt and needs to start over.

Changing for Good defines six stages of change.

- **Precontemplation.** People at this stage of change do not see that they even have a problem and will deny it when confronted. They are resisters of change, often seeing change that others can make but not the need to change themselves.

- **Contemplation.** These people are unable or uncommitted to change but are beginning to see that there is a problem and are working to understand it. If they are planning change, it is seen as in the future (six months or more).

- **Preparation.** People in this stage are planning action soon and making adjustments. They are still working to convince themselves that change is really necessary. Awareness is high at this time and planning a scheme for action is frequent.

- **Action.** This is the stage where behavior is modified. When people are working on this change, there will be changes in awareness, emotions, self-image, and thinking.

- **Maintenance.** The work of this stage of change especially centers around preventing relapse and backwards spiral in the change cycle. Note that this is not the last stage of change.

- **Termination.** This stage is the ultimate goal of change. There is no need for a continuing effort on the part of the person who has changed to be aware that the change happened. Many people never fully reach this stage.

At first glance, these stages appear linear, meaning that a person always passes sequentially from one stage to another until termination is reached. Reality is that this model is a spiral progression. The average successful self-changer recycles attempts at different stages several times before achieving ultimate success. The old adage "Two steps forward, one step back" applies to this concept. If you look at a back slide as a setback rather than a total failure, you can look at the behavior and ask yourself six questions to help you move forward with change. These questions can help you look at yourself and alter your plan for change so that you will be successful.

- What is the problem I need to solve?

- How is the problem affecting my life?

- Do I really want to change?

- How will the solution make my life different?

- How ready am I to make that change?

- What are the best strategies for me to use to be successful?

Successfully completing the journey through the progression of change is hard work. Anyone who has quit smoking can attest to that. To be successful at a change, you must develop a relapse prevention plan and intentionally continue to apply the correct processes and techniques for the stage of change you are in. Although change is difficult, the rewards are not just for your physical well-being; your mental well-being improves as much or more. Once change begins, you can feel better about yourself—you are doing it! In turn, you have taken some control back into your life.

Research about change has resulted in some interesting findings.

- Most people change by themselves, when they are ready.

- Change is not an all-or-nothing process.

- In most cases, change resembles a spiral more than a straight line.

- Efficient self-change depends on doing the right things at the right time.

- Confidence in your ability to change is the key ingredient for success.

- Feelings of self-confidence and control over your life that come from making any successful change improve your health.

(Sobel and Ornstein, p. 20.)

Two books described in this section, *Changing for Good* and *The Healthy Mind, Healthy Body Handbook* are excellent resources for helping you change. *Changing for Good* gives you examples and techniques for each stage of change and helps you to assess where you are and how you can improve your chances for change. *The Healthy Mind, Healthy Body Handbook* discusses how to accomplish many healthy behaviors by topic and why it is important to do so. As we have said, self-care habits are difficult to change, especially when they are deeply ingrained since childhood. As you read this book and find areas where you want to change, do not get discouraged if you are not successful immediately.

Chapter One
I walk down the street
There is a deep hole in the sidewalk,
I fall in.
I am lost....I am helpless.
It isn't my fault.
It takes forever to find a way out.
Chapter Two
I walk down the same street.
There is a deep hole in the sidewalk.
I pretend I don't see it.
I fall in again.
I can't believe I am in this same place.
But, it isn't my fault.
It still takes a long time to get out.
Chapter Three
I walk down the same street.
There is a deep hole in the sidewalk.
I see it is there.
I still fall in...It's a habit...but,
My eyes are open.
I know where I am.
It is my fault.
I get out immediately,
Chapter Four
I walk down the same street.
There is a deep hole in the sidewalk.
I walk around it.
Chapter Five
I walk down another street.

(There's a Hole in My Sidewalk) Portia Nelson, Hillsboro, OR: Beyond Words Publishing, Inc., 1993, pp. 2-3.

Remember that research shows that change is a spiral, but your spiral does not have to go downward. The spiral can move upward by starting again, making some changes in how you are going about the change, and then continuing until at last you reach maintenance or termination.

Portia Nelson's poem, "Autobiography in Five Short Chapters," describes the complexity of change as most of us know it.

Summary

In this chapter, we have shown you that there is a clear connection of your mind and your body. We have shown you some examples of the connection and given you the scientific background. We believe this connection is so integrated within you that the word "mindbody" might be more descriptive of the connection. Everything that happens within you **is** connected.

In Chapter Seven, "Adding Spirituality to Your Mind-Body Connection," we will take this connection a step further by describing the spiritual connection, explaining how and why the mind-body-spirit connection may be best described as a single concept.

Using your body, your mind, and your spirit, you can devise and implement the best self-care plan for you. Using your mind-body connection can help you attain your best health possible. By learning what you need to change and how to change, you can improve your quality of life, regardless of your underlying medical conditions.

The human spirit is stronger than anything that happens to it.

– Unknown

SEVEN

ADDING SPIRITUALITY TO YOUR MIND-BODY CONNECTION

*The lessons that my patients and others have learned
from personal experience are echoed in over three
hundred clinical studies that demonstrate one simple
fact: faith is good medicine.*

– Dale Matthews. M.D.

We are often asked, "How have you been able to keep going despite the difficulties of your illness?" Our first answer is often "we don't know!" However, after pausing to think about the question more deeply, we know that much of the answer lies in how we approached our own connection with God. We will be talking about how connecting to God in a way which is comfortable to you can be beneficial to your health and well-being and how you can find this connection for yourself.

Our Christian perspective has made an enormous difference in our lives. Without our faith in a loving God that we experienced in many

153

ways over the course of our illness, we know our lives would have been much more difficult. The impact of our illnesses would have been much worse and our inner strength "to get through the difficult days" would be much weaker. We would even go so far as to say that without our personal, spiritual, and religious connection we believe Carol would not be alive today.

While we are Christian and our focus in this chapter comes from our own experience with Christian practices, we do not presume to tell people who have different beliefs that their way is wrong. We hope to point you in a direction that will most help you find your spiritual connection for healing.

In the previous chapter, we discussed how your mind and body are connected and how that connection can be used to improve your life when living with chronic illness. In this chapter we will talk about spirituality and how adding it to the mind-body connection can improve and enhance health and life. Spirituality is difficult to pin down and see in scientific research, much like the interactions of the mind with the body were previously. However, studies today are showing that indeed there is a connection between the mind, the body, and the spirit. Perhaps Dr. William Salt II and Dr. Edwin H. Season have said it best:

> The intuition, experience, and scientific research attesting to the healing power of spirituality, faith, and prayer are the reasons that the concept of the mind-body connection should be expanded to include spirit. Thus, the more appropriate term is the mind-body-spirit connection. (*Fibromyalgia & the MindBodySpirit Connection* (Columbus: Parkview Publishing, 2000, p.16.)

In this chapter we will cover the following topics:

- Definitions for Understanding the Spiritual Connection

- How the Spiritual Connection May Aid Health

- Activating Your Connection

- Pushing the Activate Button to Get Connected to Your Spirituality

  - Caring Community

  - Natural Beauty

  - Ritual

- Summary

Definitions for Understanding the Spiritual Connection

In order to have a common understanding to discuss spirituality in this chapter, we will begin this chapter by giving some definitions. *God, spirituality, religion, faith, soul* and other such words are tossed around today with many different

> *He who has courage and faith will never perish in misery.*
> — Anne Frank

meanings, depending on one's personal focus. Such definitions often come from family, friends, and individual reading and experiences.

In this chapter, we will use the word *God* to encompass representative words others use for the word *God*, such as the *Divine, Creator, Higher Power,* and *Higher Self.* God is the word we have used our entire lives and are most comfortable with. You may want to fill in the word or words that you are most comfortable using and which best represents your understanding of something that is beyond you and your ability to understand. We find that friends within our Christian faith use different words to pray to God including *Holy Father, Jesus, Father in Heaven, Mother God* and many others. None of these names are right or wrong, you just need to connect and have your own name with which you are comfortable.

People often use the words *spirituality* and *religion* interchangeably. However, there are some important distinguishing characteristics. *Spirituality* refers to how a person individually orients himself or herself to God and tries to find the meaning of life. One's spirituality is private and expressed in a uniquely personal way. It gives each person a perspective with which to view life. Often spirituality is expressed to the world through religious beliefs and practices.

Religion is much less ambiguous than spirituality. Major world religions include Christianity, Judaism, Buddhism, and Islam. Religion is an orderly system of beliefs, values, symbols, and rituals used to express a group's orientation to God. A community of believers agrees upon this system. Usually your religion includes a structure for development of your own spirituality. For example, the Christian religion encourages its followers to have a personal relationship with God through Jesus Christ. Many Christians consider this personal relationship to be the cornerstone of their spirituality.

Author Dale A. Matthews, M.D., describes the similarities and differences in spirituality and religion in *The Faith Factor: Proof of the Healing Power of Prayer.* Although they are different, religion and spirituality do have two important similarities. Dr. Matthews lists these as (1) acknowledgment of the Divine and (2) teaching methods for coping with life events and emotions. (New York: Penguin Putnam Inc., 1998, pp. 182-183.)

Dr. Matthews also describes distinct differences between religion and spirituality. You may find you experience some of both religious and spiritual activities in your life. Thinking of the two sides from the list below as ends on a continuum should help you see that there can be significant differences between the definitions of religion and spirituality. The continuums should help you see that in addition to the two similarities we stated, there are significant differences between religion and spirituality.

Areas of difference between spirituality and religion fall on a continuum and examples of these differences include the following:

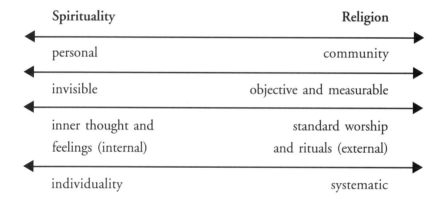

Spirituality	Religion
personal	community
invisible	objective and measurable
inner thought and feelings (internal)	standard worship and rituals (external)
individuality	systematic

You most likely experience parts of all of these on both sides of the continuum and in-between. The continuums are to show the extreme ends of each so you can examine where you are.

You have within you the essence of which you were created to be. Your *soul* is that kernel deep within you that is who you are, your essence. Your soul is your connection back to the Divine. Jean Shinola Bolen, M.D., describes illness as "a profound soul event." She says, "Illness is both soul-shaking and soul-evoking for the patient and for all others for whom the patient matters." (*Close to the Bone: Life Threatening Illness and the Search for Meaning*, New York: Simon & Schuster, 1996 p. 14.)

> *Now faith is being sure of what we hope for and certain of what we do not see.*
>
> – Hebrews 11:1, New International Version

Perhaps your own soul has been thoroughly shaken by your illness. Your illness may get you in better touch with your soul, true self, and your purpose. In this chapter, we will talk about how you can connect with your soul to improve your life with chronic illness. In the following chapter we will talk about how illness affects your purpose.

Faith and *belief* are often used alongside *religion, spirituality,* and *soul.* One way to describe *faith* is that it is based on trusting things that are invisible, or believing without proof. In 1910 William Osler, a Canadian physician, described faith as "the one great moving force which we can neither weigh in balance nor test in the crucible." Faith cannot be measured or proven in any logical way. Faith goes a step beyond *belief.* Usually we believe something because we have seen proof and became convinced that there is enough proof to believe. Faith, on the other hand, includes a belief in something, even if it is immeasurable. There is an unexplainable devotion and trust that surrounds a person's faith. No logical argument can easily change the mind of a person with faith. As our son Eric puts it, "Faith is just that, faith."

When you are practicing your faith, you are putting your trust in something or someone. Faith has been creatively expressed in different ways over the years. Theologians talk about faith in many ways. Nineteenth century Danish philosopher Soren Kierkegaard describes faith as a "leap." In the movie *Indiana Jones and the Last Crusade,* Indiana takes a giant step of faith in his search for the Holy Grail. As he steps (leaps) out across the dark abyss below him, a bridge appears from nowhere to carry him to safety. That is how it is with faith; it provides an invisible bridge to carry you safely across the territory of your life-changing illness.

Within a Christian context faith gives purpose and meaning while you are here on earth and belief for a life after death. The Bible describes faith as "being sure of what we hope for and certain of what we do not see." (Hebrews 11:1, New International Version.) Purpose, meaning and hope are bridges to living better with life-changing illness.

The words *belief* and *faith* are not just used within the context of religion. In the last chapter we described how Dr. Herbert Benson has studied the role of faith in the healing process. Dr. Benson believes that the brain is "wired for beliefs and expectancies. When activated, the body can respond as it would if the belief were reality." (*Timeless Healing: The Power and Biology of Belief,* New York: Scribner, 1996, p. 63.) A simple example outside of the spiritual/religious context is the following. Your reaction of faith and belief can be seen in the simple example of watching a scary movie with spooky music and special effects. You will generally experience physical effects as if the story on the screen were actually happening. Your hands may be clammy, your heart may beat faster, you may be holding your breath, or having other physical reactions. The music and special effects trick your mind into the false belief that something scary is about to happen.

When you have faith in a loving God, your mind's response can have physical reactions, thus contributing to positive changes. This physical benefit can be seen with spiritually uplifting music. Many people would confirm that a sad mood can be lifted with spiritual

> *Light is to the painter what faith is to humankind.*
>
> – Herbert Benson, M.D.

music. This music may include old time gospel, hymns, contemporary Christian, and new age style of soothing music. Dr. Benson describes "wiring" for belief as being within each of us. When you activate this wiring with spirituality and faith, rather than fear and disbelief as in the above paragraph, you can change your body's physical and emotional response. The person with health and optimism may renew his body to a healthier state.

How the Spiritual Connection May Aid Health

Many researchers have tried to explain how and why spirituality and faith connect to better health results. There are certain inherent problems with scientifically measuring spirituality and faith and their effect on your health. Because *spirituality* and *faith* are such nebulous words, putting a religious structure around them enables the effects of spirituality and faith to be studied and measured scientifically.

Religion is much more concrete than *spirituality* or *faith*. Looking at a specific religion or a denomination's faith practices helps researchers to learn about how people within a specific group understand a supreme life meaning. Researchers then are able to use worshippers of a specific religious group to study their religion as a factor in health and healing. By studying the effect of faith in the context of a specific religious group or denomination, scientists have been able to see how faith connects to the mind and body and to health and healing.

Science has shown that one's religion, spirituality, and health are closely associated. For the reasons stated previously, scientifically proving that religion caused the improvement is difficult. Religion is definitely a factor that affects our health along with factors such as gender, race, age, and health practices. Most people who actively practice religion and/or spirituality believe that spirituality has a causal role in their mental and physical well-being.

The spiritual connection, activated within a religious context, can be beneficial to your health. Some of these health and life benefits include:

- You may heal faster and with fewer complications if you develop a serious illness.

- You may have a longer life expectancy.

- You cope with peacefulness and experience less pain when your life is threatened by serious or terminal illness.

- People with religious involvement tend to steer clear of problems with alcohol, drugs, and tobacco.

- You enjoy a more stable marriage and family life.

- You find a greater sense of meaning and purpose in your life.

Imagine a prescription of spirituality that offers you tremendous health benefits and has virtually no negative side effects! Some doctors are beginning to believe that religious or spiritual involvement should be a part of each patient's treatment plan.

Science has shown people can prevent illness, recover from illness, and—most remarkably—live longer when they find ways to connect with their spirituality. The more you connect, the more likely you are to benefit. Despite the positive healing effects and comparatively low side effects, doctors usually say little or nothing to patients about the health benefits of spirituality. We believe this is largely due to the lack of training doctors receive regarding considering this important aspect in their patient exams. Many doctors are uncomfortable discussing this topic with patients. With this in mind, you may want to tell your doctor how spirituality affects your life.

We want you to remember that although you can improve your life in many ways by using the faith factor as a personal prescription, there are several important concepts that can play into your spiritual connection.

- **Death.** No one has conquered death in this world. Everyone still dies sometime. As Dr. Joan Borysenko reminded us in the previous chapter, even the most spiritual and religiously faithful people have suffered from disease or illness and eventually died. Mother Teresa, Joan of Arc, St. Francis of Assissi, and other saints and strong believers still are human and every human eventually meets the same fate—our earthly bodies die.

- **Unhealthy religion or toxic spirituality.** When the religion or the religious community that surrounds you is unhealthy, there are negative side effects that deter the healthy benefits of the faith factor. Here are two examples:

  - A belief system that holds that your illness was directly and only caused by sin.

  - A belief that if you follow a specific, prescribed regimen, such as a proper way to pray, you will be healed.

  Either one of these beliefs can easily lead you to feel like you did something wrong or you wouldn't have gotten sick or you would be healed by now. As a result, you can get down on yourself, disappointed that you didn't "do it" better. Playing such a blame game works against your healing process.

  Unhealthy or toxic beliefs are not always easy to recognize. A good guideline to follow is that if practicing those beliefs makes you feel uncomfortable or as if you have no choice regarding your actions and beliefs, then there may be some toxic characteristics.

- **Unknown results.** The kind of healing that takes place in your body, mind, and spirit can come in many shapes, sizes, and time lines. This is very important to remember as you use your spiritual practices to promote healing. When you practice spirituality, there is a basis for you to have a very high expectation of complete healing. Unfortunately, this does not always happen. Why some people have dramatic healing experiences and others do not goes unexplained. When Carol gets to heaven, one of her first questions for God will be, "Why do some people suffer while others do not?" (Unfortunately, if she gets there before you, you may have to wait your turn for the answer to this and other profound questions because there is no easy way that we know of to transmit this insightful information back to those on earth.)

With that said, actively practicing your faith and connecting to your spirituality have tremendous benefits and can be a very important part of your formula for healing.

Activating Your Connection

As we discussed in the prior chapter, your mind's thoughts are connected to your body's neurochemicals, with far-reaching physical effects throughout your body. A person who has a spiritual connection to God and/or the infinite is likely to feel greater comfort, solace, and safety than someone who does not exercise this connection. An important question to answer is how can we activate our connection to God, Higher Self or the Infinite with our own inner soul and spirit. Later in this chapter we will share several ways that we have learned to connect.

Dr. Matthews and Dr. Benson (along with a growing number of other physicians) are advocates of integrating a patient's spiritual practices into their treatment plans. Dr. Matthews suggests, based on research, that when resources of a patient's faith are linked with the resources of medicine, people often get better faster, get better unexpectedly, and cope better with remaining symptoms.

> *Spiritual growth is honed and perfected only through practice. Like an instrument, it must be played. Like a path, it must be walked.*
>
> – Kent Nerburn

There are many spiritual healing practices. These may include prayer, meditation, centering prayer, relaxation, imagery, reading scripture, healthy lifestyles, and religious community support.

Casual observation and serious research have shown that people who practice religion fall into one of two categories. There are those who are either intrinsic or extrinsic followers of their religion.

- **Intrinsic followers.** Intrinsic followers "walk the talk." In other words, what they say and do during the week fits what they do when they are seen practicing their religion in worship. They are motivated by a deep faith that is right for their soul. They work to help their fellow man for no earthly reward. Their practices fit the definition of *spirituality* as well as *religion.*

- **Extrinsic followers.** Extrinsic followers are the ones that use their religious practices for another end, such as power, control, social and business status, etc. They have not bought into their religious practices on a soul level.

Research has shown that intrinsic followers are more likely to benefit from their religious beliefs and practices. To receive the benefits of a faith factor prescription, intrinsic belief is necessary. It is not possible to go through the motions of practicing a religion if that is all you are doing. In other words, the deep connection and devotional faith to God and the Divine is that which can help people heal. (Matthews, pp. 54-55.)

Pushing the Activate Button to Get Connected to Your Spirituality

The following are several areas where we have personally been able to see and receive benefit from the healing connection by using our spirituality and religion. We have chosen to look at several facets of spirituality and faith, sharing with you a few of our personal experiences. We hope these stories will help you connect to your own personal experiences so that you can be motivated to practice them and connect to the health benefits that are being attributed to them. Your "activate buttons" include caring community, natural beauty, and ritual.

Caring Community

When we think of the people who have reached out to help us, we feel a deep sense of support and peace. From the earliest days of Carol's illness and later with Doug's illness, many supportive people have surrounded us. These people helped us through our darkest days. They were the bridge that carried us across many deep abysses of fear, where we sometimes felt inadequate to "keep going."

When people wonder what they can do to help someone, Carol suggests simply asking the person who needs help what he or she needs. If possible, make specific suggestions rather than asking in a general way. People who were helpful to us said, "I'm going to the grocery, what do you need?," "I would like to have your child over this afternoon, can he come?," "Please come over to our place for dinner with us," or "I made an extra meat loaf tonight and would like to know when to bring it over." We have found offers of specific assistance much easier to accept than vague offers like, "How I can help?" We learned to accept these offers graciously, as it not only helped whoever was sick but also the rest of the family. Our family, often including our mothers, had a burden lifted for the moment. Usually the load lifted was much greater than the immediate service or need that was filled.

Our couples group at church literally picked us up in the early days of Carol's illness when Eric was a preschooler, by doing everything from baby-sitting to grocery shopping to toilet cleaning and laundry. Their practical help was great, but the knowledge that friends cared and were holding us in prayer was even better. The same went for our families, especially our parents, aunts and uncles and brothers. Everyone helped at one time or another in various capacities. It not only gave us emotional and physical support, it gave our son some stability in what was a very chaotic time in our family. Another friend, who was part of a small group of friends we had known since school, took Eric to her home any day Carol needed extra rest, even on short notice. She also wrote Carol notes she called "Susie's Newsies" every day Carol was in the hospital (nine hospital stays in 18 months). Those notes brought untold uplifting of Carol's soul and she knew she could count on them during very dark hospital days.

We mentioned earlier that we believe we would not be here without our spiritual connection. Part of that connection came through the many prayers that were prayed on our behalf. In 1988, Carol had three cardiac arrests due to a pacemaker wire's failure. The third arrest happened while she was being observed in a hospital intensive care unit. Carol was unstable and unconscious for about an hour. When she regained consciousness, she learned that her husband, mother, a minister, and several devoted friends were waiting. We have no doubt these friends prayed Carol through a time that her cardiologist called "a miracle."

Community can benefit you in many ways. Be open to people's caring words and deeds. Soak them in like a sponge and learn to draw on the nourishment of your community, friends, and family for the dark days of your illness. In experiencing community of this kind, you are also experiencing other faith remedies. One is the ritual of unexpected help. For almost a year early in Carol's illness, Doug's brother and sister-in-law brought dinner and ate with us on Wednesday nights. The unity of people coming together with a common cause and mutual trust and allowing others to do tasks that you once thought only you could do for yourself, are all part of activating spirituality's healing benefits.

Natural Beauty

Beauty comes in many forms that touch the senses. Sounds include music and nature sounds such as birds, rain, ocean or wind rustling through the trees. Sights include immense sights as mountains or oceans and more everyday sights as sunshine, flowers, and perhaps rainbows. Smells and tastes include favorite foods and flowers. Touch may include feeling a warm breeze or cold snow flakes on your nose.

One place to experience beauty is in a worship sanctuary. Beauty in a church can include stained glass windows, sacred music, quiet, liturgical art and sometimes scents such as incense. The great cathedrals of Europe invoke within us a feeling of beauty, adoration, and awe that are truly a feast for eyes and ears. Other forms of beauty are no different in evoking a sense of awe and power beyond ourselves.

The Creator, who is greater than any of us, created all of these experiences. By noticing and enjoying the beauty of your world you can remind yourself that there is a larger meaning for you and for your world to focus on. Noticing beauty helps you sense a higher purpose that is positive, loving, and capable of creating beauty. It takes you outside of yourself, connecting you to your God, Creator, or Higher Power.

Ritual

When you do the same thing over and over, like your routine at home or prescribed religious rituals, you tend to have a feeling of continuity and safety. Rituals are comfortable because you know what to expect.

> *Belief in God lends us a will to live we would not have without God.*
>
> – Herbert Benson, M.D.

While you deal with life-changing illness, knowing there are constants in life can be very reassuring. Rituals can be experienced daily. Prayers at mealtime, perhaps even the same prayer you said when you were a child, bedtime prayers, repetition of soothing Bible verses, or using a relaxation or meditation practice can be health giving. Ancient Jewish rituals include the Sabbath dinner and Passover. Prayers have been used for thousands of years. Another ancient ritual practice still in use is the Rosary Prayer practiced by Roman Catholics.

Summary

This chapter has explored the meaning of spirituality and suggested that spirituality is a personal yet powerful ally in dealing with all aspects of life, especially for people dealing with life-changing illness. You also saw how you can use your spiritual connection as an essential prescription for living with life-changing illness, with no harmful side effects.

Margaret Baim, M.S., R.N., C.S., from Harvard's Mind/Body Medical Institute, says, "Healing transcends the physical by engaging your spirit's expression to influence your thoughts, emotions and actions. The healer is truly within, and cultivates a strong relationship with one's own spiritual nature, which is the quintessential mind/body interaction."

As you incorporate your own methods to make this connection in your daily life, you will begin to have a greater and greater effect on your health. As you get more in touch with and find ways to deepen your understanding of the infinite, your spiritual life will have a positive impact on your health in your mind, body, and spirit.

Serious, life-changing illness may totally change many aspects of your life. It may change your occupation, affect your interactions with others, and redefine the place of spirituality in your life—how you connect with God. Many people with an illness struggle to find these connections, how to define success in their lives and how to find activities that are rewarding. These issues, which are key components of defining your purpose, are discussed in the next chapter.

The concept of the mind-body connection should be expanded to include spirit. Thus, the more appropriate term is the mind-body-spirit connection.

– William B. Salt II, M.D. and
Edwin H. Season, M.D.

EIGHT

FINDING YOUR PURPOSE IN THE MIDST OF PAIN

to be nobody but yourself—in a world which
is doing its best, night and day, to make you
everybody else—means to fight the hardest battle
which any human being can fight,
and never stop fighting.

— e.e. cummings

W hy am I here, what can I do that is worthwhile, now that my life has been turned upside down? We have both asked, cried, and even screamed out these questions at various times throughout our illnesses. Many people ask similar questions when faced with illness, particularly a serious illness. These questions are the focus of this chapter. We will also look at learning what strengths, talents, and gifts you have to offer in spite of your illness.

As we discussed in Chapter One, illness often presents a crisis that turns your life upside down. We described crisis in terms of the Chinese word for crisis, which is a combination of the symbols for danger and opportunity. Life-changing illness gives you the opportunity to develop a new sense of who you are and to rediscover your purpose in life. In *The Power of Purpose: Creating Meaning in Your Life and Work,* author Richard J. Leider says, "Crisis is the mirror of purpose. Crisis brings us face to face with the big questions." (San Francisco: Barrett-Koehler, 1997, p. 7.) A mirror brings you face-to-face with yourself. A crisis brings you face-to-face with yourself. You suddenly have an opportunity within the challenge of illness to look again at what is really important to you.

A serious, life-changing illness may totally change many facets of your life. It may change your occupation, affect your interactions with others, and redefine the place of spirituality in your life—how you connect with God. Many people with an illness struggle with how to find these connections, how to define success in one's life, and how to find rewarding activity. These issues are key components of defining your purpose.

Your illness may force you to view your approach to life in a different way than healthy people do. You may be defining your purpose for the first time or from a totally new perspective. This chapter will focus on topics which address the basic questions, "Why am I here and what is my purpose?"

- A Definition of Purpose

- Are You Living Your Life On Accident or On Purpose?

  - Living On Accident

  - Living On Purpose

- Defining Your Purpose

- Energy Expenditures

- Questions We Ask When We Make a Decision

- Life Is a Journey, Not a Destination

- Summary

A Definition of Purpose

Author Richard J. Leider says, "Purpose is that deepest dimension within us—our central core or essence—where we have a profound sense of who we are, where we came from, and where we're going. Purpose is the quality around which we choose to shape our lives. Purpose is a source of energy and direction." (Leider, p. 30.) We especially like the phrase *source of energy* for describing purpose. Those of us with life-changing illness are often tired (Carol's word is exhausted!), so being able to find a source for tapping into energy sounds very helpful. As you look into purpose as a tool to use for changing how you now live your life, remember that it may be a key to unlocking an inner energy for living.

> *Learn what you are, and be such.*
>
> – Pindar

Are You Living Your Life On Accident or On Purpose?

Many people today go through life constantly busy. They are running everywhere but do not know their destination. Busyness is often seen as an admirable trait in our world today. Has anyone asked you how you are, and you answer "Busy!"? In our society, being busy suggests you are important, your life is worth living. Busyness is a mark of success. However, what is being accomplished with this busyness of today's lifestyle? On-accident living is very often a part of this busy lifestyle.

Sometimes you may need to assess why you have been so busy. As you learn to live with your life-changing illness, you may realize for the first time that you need to live differently. You may begin to question whether you are living on purpose or on accident? You may wonder what you can do to make life easier.

> *There is just one life for each of us: our own.*
>
> – Euripides

When you practice on-purpose living, you think through what you value and make choices about what you do and how you live your life. Those values become your new basis for making decisions.

Living On Accident

If you simply take life as it comes, disorganized and drifting without a map, you are most likely living life on accident. You may be busy simply because there doesn't seem to be any other way to get the job done. Living a busy life as an on-accident person, by putting your health and yourself in the back seat and by letting your life control you, may be hazardous to your health at any time but especially when you have a life-changing illness.

Besides drifting about, people who live life on accident often find themselves too busy, or put another way, "in over their heads." Literally, the phrase "in over your head" refers to being in water over your head. When you are in deep water, it becomes very hard work just to swim in place and stay above water. In our example, the water is your busy life. Life often becomes "deep water" and difficult even when you are not sick. However, as you are probably well aware, when you have an illness, the water of your life gets deeper much faster and becomes much harder to tread. Sometimes this makes your illness worse. Many times Carol has had to make decisions based on what was most important and how her health would be affected. Being too busy affected her health and her ability to do important activities.

Before your illness, there were probably times when you felt like you were living life "in over your head," trying to maintain an unplanned and often overcommitted agenda. You may have been too tired, made mistakes, become depressed, and been very irritable. People may have told you how miserable you were to be around. These reactions to living an on-accident life are often warning signs. Your body was probably telling you that your lifestyle could be leading you toward problems. When you were healthy, you probably had the physical resiliency to "manage," even if you were not taking care of yourself very well. The ability to get by with doing too much usually is lost if you suffer with life-changing illness.

> *You've got to be very careful if you don't know where you are going, because you might not get there.*
>
> – Yogi Berra

Your body is not a silent partner when you abuse it by living an on-accident lifestyle. Your body speaks to you all the time. However, most people do not listen to their bodies or understand their bodies' language. Your body speaks when it is thirsty by saying, "My mouth is dry." It is speaking to you in the only language it knows, "I need water." Your body speaks when it is hot by perspiring; it is saying, "I need to find a cool spot to sit down for a while." Listening to your body becomes more important with illness because even under your best circumstances you are fighting an uphill battle. Living life on purpose gives you another option, an entirely different way to live life.

Living On Purpose

As the words "on purpose" imply, on-purpose living means you make intentional choices about what you do and how you do it. On-purpose living has some specific characteristics.

- You know your purpose

- You listen to your body and accept your limits

- You have a vision of your future

- You direct your life accordingly

Accepting and following this four-part prescription for on-purpose living may help you turn your life around. We are not saying that on-purpose living will make you well. We do believe, however, that you are certain to make your life easier, more rewarding, and more enjoyable. As we said at the beginning of the chapter, living on purpose can be energizing. Using this approach will create a new set of lenses through which you see your life. With these new lenses you will see yourself as a valuable person despite whatever the specific limitations your life-changing illness has given you. You and your purpose will now look different in the "crisis mirror."

Whether your pain is the emotional pain of detoured plans or physical pain of illness, if you do not have a reason for being or can no longer perform in life as you did before, you may feel as if life has no meaning. Some people who feel this way then choose to remain in this void and become stagnant, depressed, afraid, or angry. Life can seem futile and almost unbearable. If you have these feelings, be assured you are not alone. These depressed feelings are a part of adjusting to illness. You are adjusting to the loss of being able to perform in life as you did before.

If finding a special purpose seems ridiculous at this time, then think of just finding a purpose for today. At the end of the day look back and see how you made a difference today. Did you cheer someone up, call a friend, feed the birds,

> *Having a goal is a state of happiness.*
>
> – E.J. Bartek

smile to a stranger? These activities and many other simple activities make a difference in your life. Tomorrow do the same thing. Taking things one day at a time can be essential for living on purpose with life-changing illness.

You may be familiar with the story of professional golfer Casey Martin, whose rare circulatory system ailment limits his ability to walk. His highly visible, well-publicized challenge of the Professional Golfers Association to allow him to use a cart in the PGA tournaments has raised the public attention to the fact that golfers who are highly skilled but have physical challenges may deserve to have the right to play golf with a cart. Martin knows that he has a limited number of years where his health will permit him to play competitive golf, even with a cart. He knows his purpose— to play on the PGA tour—which has empowered him to take on a very difficult challenge.

Defining Your Purpose

When you define and become aware of your specific purpose, you can develop a more positive outlook and be energized mentally and physically. You can have a better sense of your value as a person.

A good purpose statement for living does not need to be complicated or difficult to remember. It does not need to require physical energy which you may not have. However, the statement is the core of your being. It is the soul or essence of who you are. You may already have one

> *When I can get people to accept themselves as whole individuals, lovable as they are, they become able to give from an inner strength.*
>
> – Bernie Siegel, M.D.

that you try to live but not realize it. A good purpose statement can be very short and simple. If you are able to identify your purpose and label it, remembering your purpose on a daily basis will be easier. It will help you to write your purpose on your heart in order that you may live it.

Here is another way to look at purpose. A good purpose statement is like a brochure or postcard of your trip's destination. This trip has a road hazard of life-changing illness. The illness dictates which roads and choices you make. With a purpose, a destination, you know where you eventually want to be. You make adjustments for the illness (as with a road hazard or detour), but you can still get where you are going (your purpose).

If you do not know where you are going, how can you get there? Instead, if you do know where your destination is, you can develop a map to get there. The route to your goal may be different because of illness, but the end result can be the same.

We have had to change the route to our goals several times. Before his illness, Doug clearly saw his professional career as a partner with a major international consulting firm as an important mission in his life. Carol clearly saw being a wife and mother as an important mission in her life. Being a nurturing wife and mother (which meant caring for Doug's and Eric's needs) seemed like a very appropriate goal for her when she was 25 years old with an 18-month-old child in 1979.

When life-changing illness comes along in your life, "stuff happens" and the crisis mirror reflects your need to change assumptions about how to accomplish your purpose. You may even realize that you need a totally different purpose for your life. You and the world around you may look different in the mirror with your life-changing illness. Carol remembers a time when she had to challenge these assumptions and describes it below:

> I needed to take an entirely new look at what motherhood meant and revise that role and my goals to fit my new reality. Suddenly, being the best mother meant arranging the best care for Eric when I was hospitalized or too sick to care for him by myself.
>
> Being a good mother could not mean dressing like June Cleaver, the perfect housewife and mother from the 1950's television show "Leave it to Beaver," vacuuming and dusting the house three times a day to maintain an immaculate house and fixing perfect Betty Crocker meals. However, being mother could and did include making a ritual of reading naptime and bedtime stories to Eric, my preschool son. This was something I could do no matter how sick I was. Being mother also meant learning how to accept help from outsiders to make life better for Eric. Such help included accepting rides to preschool from others and accepting opportunities for him to go to play groups even when I could not attend. Seeing gracious acceptance of help as a part of my role as a nurturing mother was not "giving in" to my illness. Rather it was realigning my purpose and thoughts to see this as empowering me to do the best job I could as a mother.
>
> Was this easy? No way! Did I know that what I was doing at the time was living my purpose? Only partially. I remember viewing those who helped with Eric as his special angels. I got by with more than "a little help from my friends." Looking back I can see how this was realigning my goals to accomplish my mission or purpose at that time. I could still be a good mother even with life-changing illness. The route to being a nurturing mother was different, but I think I still was able to accomplish that purpose.

Life-changing illness requires you to take a whole new look at who you are, why you are here and how you will accomplish your goals. Regularly and creatively re-examining your mission and purpose is essential to leading an on-purpose life that is aligned with good self-care.

What is your story? Isak Dinesen said, "God made man because he loved stories." What will your story be and how will you or others know you are living it? What will the pictures look like in your storybook? In other words, what would living your purpose look like if you were watching it being lived out by you on a television show? What would you be doing? Thinking of your purpose in action words may be a more concrete way for some to understand their purpose.

Following are some resources that might be useful for you in sorting out your purpose, mission and story.

- Laurie Beth Jones' *The Path: Creating Your Mission Statement for Work and for Life* is a helpful resource, including a book and accompanying workbook to help you find your mission and purpose. (Hyperion, 1998.) Although the book does not specifically address purpose in relation to illness, it is still a helpful resource. This book and her other resources can be found at www.lauriebethjones.com. You can create a mission statement on her Web site at www.lauriebethjones.com/mission.

- www.franklincovey.com/customer/missionform.html is a Web site offering a convenient way to work quickly through a mission statement, making the process both fun and easy. You can come up with something about yourself that may be just what you need to refocus, or at least you can get a very good start.

- Another well written book mentioned in this chapter is *The Power of Purpose: Creating Meaning in Your Life and Work* by Richard J. Leider (San Francisco: Barrett-Koehler, 1997). He has studied what older people wish they had done more of. Leider does an excellent job of relating purpose to life and career.

Energy Expenditures

Once you know what your purpose is, you will begin to naturally ask yourself, "Is this project or event worthwhile for me to be doing?" and "Does it help fulfill my purpose?" That

> *Purpose is a source of energy and direction.*
>
> Richard J. Leider

doesn't need to mean that it is not important. It simply means rather that the project, event, or detail does not need to take up *your* scarce time and energy. In other words, doing it yourself may not enhance your life at this time.

Remember, your purpose statement does not need to be complicated. Just because your purpose statement is short does not mean it is not important. Mother Theresa's mission statement was very short, "To show mercy and compassion to the dying." She lived out her mission statement one act at a time for her whole life, even when she was quite ill. By doing so, she touched millions of lives, directly or indirectly. By living a simple purpose statement, Mother Theresa was able to have the statement *written in her heart* so that she could easily remember it daily, or more likely moment to moment.

One way you might think about activities and events is to view them as energy expenditures. An energy expenditure is something that uses up energy. A 500-mile car trip might burn up 20 or more gallons of gasoline. A two-hour homeowners' association committee meeting might use up all of your available energy, energy you might otherwise have used to do something really important, like getting adequate rest, doing your job, or spending time with your spouse or children.

Keeping yourself healthy and quickly distinguishing between healthy and unhealthy energy expenditures are new concepts for most people.

We suggest that you ask yourself the following question, *"Does this activity fit my purpose and keep me as healthy as possible?"* The busy world drives you in many directions that are not always of your own choosing. Now that you face life-changing illness, knowing your purpose and letting your own purpose drive you become even more important than before you were ill. You no longer have a reserve tank of energy.

When you have a life-changing illness, maintaining your health becomes your number one purpose. This purpose influences every other purpose you have. We imagine that Mother Theresa frequently asked herself, "Does this activity help my purpose of showing mercy and compassion to the dying?" She appeared to have endless energy, most likely because all of her energy was spent accomplishing her life purpose, minimizing needless drains of energy as a result of extraneous activities.

Questions We Ask When We Make a Decision

When we are asked to take on a project, deciding whether or not to buy something, going on a vacation, doing a group activity, or other activities, we try to ask ourselves a few questions before we get to an answer of "yes" or "no." First, we ask

1. *Will it simplify our lives?*

2. *Is it a worthwhile and important activity (regardless of who does it)?*

3. *Does it fit our personal purpose statements?*

4. *Is it good self-care for our health while living with an illness?*

If the answer is "yes," we are likely to say "yes" to the activity or project. If it does not simplify our lives, then we ask ourselves three more questions to determine if we should expend the energy that the activity will take.

If we answer "no" to any of these questions, we know we should probably say "no" to the activity. Even if we answer "yes" to the first three questions, if the answer to the health question is "no," we try to find another way for the activity to be accomplished. Neither of us would say it is easy or that we make appropriate decisions all the time, but asking these questions helps us sort and plan our lives within our limits. Several times we have had a vacation trip planned, only to realize that the effort of getting ready, getting there, intensively "relaxing," returning home, and re-entering to our routine wasn't going to pass our four-question test. We canceled our reservations and took a vacation at home but told very few people about our change of plans.

Finally, we ask

5. *Have we slept on it?*

We have discovered that we don't need to answer "yes" or "no" immediately. We almost always ask for some time, even if it's just overnight, to "sleep on it." "Buying time" like this gives us time to work through the other four questions described above. Our hearts may be saying "yes," but our minds need time to process the data and answer "yes" or "no" appropriately.

Life Is a Journey, Not a Destination

Life is a marathon, not a sprint. Life-changing illness can make life feel like an uphill run with a 17 mile per hour head wind and one leg in a cast.

The idea of life as a journey, rather than a destination, may sound unfamiliar. Most of us tend to focus on our destination. We have pointed out earlier that you need to know where you are going and what you want from your life. Your life-changing illness gives your journey a new context. It may even change your destination and your purpose. But the journey is sometimes the best part of life.

Think for a moment about a plane ride for a business trip. There is a specific place where the business traveler is headed and a specific job to be done when the traveler gets there. But consciously stopping to enjoy the billowing clouds, blue skies, and beautiful mountain ranges during the flight can be great, too. Enjoying the journey means putting aside for a moment thinking about your destination and enjoying the moment, not wanting to miss seeing the clouds around you or the mountains below.

When you have an illness, you especially need to watch the terrain as you go. When you are ill, it helps more than ever before to enjoy the small things along the way. Enjoying the journey helps you to look beyond yourself.

All of us are human beings, not just human doings! As a very young child, Doug thought we were human "beans." Sometimes we do feel like Mexican jumping beans, moving around faster and faster and enjoying it less and less. In Chapter Six, we discussed a relaxation response exercise called mindfulness, the attitude of being mindful and present in the moment. Mindfulness allows you to be aware of what you are doing, why you are doing it, and how the action is affecting you. By just being, you can remember to take care of yourself, enjoy the little things, and make choices that fit your new lifestyle. By slowing down you can make healthy choices and bring back a balance and focus to your life that is by your choice, not a choice driven by human doings. So, don't just do something, sit there!

Summary

On-purpose living can change your life in a very positive way. We don't want to imply that knowing who you are and knowing your purpose are easily decided one-time events. They evolve and change over time, whether you are healthy or deal with chronic, life-changing illness. With chronic illness there is an even greater need to look at yourself because of the greater limits imposed by your illness. Taking care of your health takes on a prominent role and must be your first priority. Living with awareness of your purpose, what you need and want to do, and staying within the limitations of your illness can be a new, healthier way to live. Sometimes, this requires you to realign your attitude, as discussed in the next chapter.

Be what you are—that is the only thing one can ask of anybody.

– Paul Tillich

NINE

REALIGNING YOUR ATTITUDE

People are just as happy as they make up their minds to be.

– Abraham Lincoln

*D*o you sometimes wonder why you are so upset, frustrated or angry? Can you change your attitude? Do you think of "having an attitude" as something negative? These are some of the questions people tend to ask when they wrestle with attitude.

People often look at thoughts or attitudes of themselves and others as being uncontrollable, a claim that Abraham Lincoln argued against. His statement about people being as happy as they make up their minds to be certainly has a lot of truth, but it doesn't tell the whole story. Sometimes it is extremely difficult to "make up" your mind to be happy. Lincoln must have known that firsthand, because he suffered from severe depression.

When someone is irritable or disagreeable, you might say that person has a "bad attitude." Another widely used expression is, "She sure has an attitude today!" As you can see, neither use of attitude here is positive. The general connotation of the word is negative. Even our chapter title talks about changing or realigning your attitude, implying that your attitude is negative or bad.

However, your attitude can be positive. Your attitude can help you make the best of a bad situation. This does not mean your more negative attitudes need to hide as if nothing has changed in your life. You do need to allow yourself to look realistically at the impact of changes in your life brought about by your illness. Many aspects of your life may have changed because of your illness. These changes may cause you disappointments, heartache, and grief. We are not asking you to ignore these feelings. Understanding and acknowledging those feelings is quite healthy.

Attitudes are not cast in concrete. You can change yours. Converting negative thoughts and attitudes into positive ones is safe and effective therapy, with no known adverse side effects. Research has shown that your attitude is healthiest when it is realistic, hopeful, and filled with humor. We hope this chapter will help you see what you can do to realign your attitude towards a healthier outlook.

In this chapter, we will discuss the following topics:

- Analyzing Your Attitude

- Brain Chemistry and Attitude

- How Medication Can Promote a Healthy Attitude

- Attitudes, Actions, and Beliefs

- Recognizing Beliefs that Strangle a Healthy Attitude

- Methods to Analyze Attitude

- Attitude Tapes

- Developing a Stress-Hardy Attitude

- Writing to Clear Out Your Brain's Cobwebs

- Humor for Health

- Summary

Analyzing Your Attitude

The previous chapter discussed how understanding your purpose can help you change the choices you make. A healthy attitude can also change your choices. Your attitude dramatically influences how you view yourself, your illness, and your changed life. Although this is not always easy to see, a healthy attitude can help you open your eyes to the positive side of your illness in the midst of changes to your lifestyle.

> *Man is not disturbed by events, but by the view he takes of them.*
>
> – Epictetus

The World Book Dictionary defines attitude as "a way of thinking, acting, or feeling; feeling, manner, or behavior of a person toward a situation or cause." (*The World Book Dictionary*, New York: World Book, Inc. Publishing, 1989, p. 132.) It is interesting that the definition uses all three words (thinking, acting, feeling) because psychologists debate among themselves which comes first: how you think, how you feel, or what you do.

Psychologist Alice Domar, Director of the Mind/Body Center for Women's Health at Harvard Medical School's Mind/Body Medical Institute, shares the following riddle when she talks to patients about changing their attitudes. See if you can guess the answer before you see the answer that is revealed.

Goose in the Bottle: A Riddle for Our Times

Imagine that you have in front of you a large glass bottle that contains a large, healthy, and happy goose. How can you get that goose out of the bottle, without either breaking the bottle or harming the goose?

Are you stuck? Here's a hint. You are approaching the problem too concretely.

Are you still stuck? Another hint: Ask yourself how the goose got in the bottle in the first place.

****

The answer to this question, which you may have spent several minutes pondering, can be found in the initial posing of the riddle. Since you are only asked to imagine the goose in the bottle, all you need to do is remove the goose in your imagination. Imagine the goose in; imagine the goose out.

This riddle makes a point that I drive home to my patients: many of our everyday worries are as illusory as that goose in the bottle. We imagine inescapable traps that are nothing more than figments of our worst fantasies. The goose-in-the-bottle exercise illustrates that many of our problems can be solved when we realize that our minds are creating them – and our minds can undo them.

(Reprinted with permission from Harvard Medical School's Mind/ Body Medical Institute.)

Many people find it hard to think outside the box, or outside the bottle! Yet just one thought, whether true or false, can totally change how you look at your situation.

For example, our friend Sharon initially looked at her back injury as a life-long sentence of immobilizing pain. With the help of a mental health counselor, Sharon was able to rethink her attitude about her situation. When she reevaluated her pain (her goose in the bottle) she realized that there were methods to tackle the pain that she had not known about. She learned new ways of sitting and standing to relieve the stress on her back muscles. She learned to use an imagery tape for 20 minutes every afternoon during the time of day when her pain was at its worst. She learned to do minis throughout her day to refocus her mind away from the pain. She began to take time for herself, something she had not done for a long time. She began to take short walks as her back would allow, soaking in the sun, and listening to the birds sing and the breeze blow through the trees. These activities helped Sharon find a new attitude about her back pain. She was able to reshape her attitude. She no longer saw herself as a person defined only by her back pain, but as someone with some control over her daily life decisions which affect her level of pain. She has learned that it is important to take care of herself. She still has pain from time to time, but she knows she can make choices to help decrease her pain.

Look at your basic view of illness. Everyone views it differently. Many of these differences are based on one's own life experience. People's unique, personal experience greatly affects how they react when faced with a life-changing

> *Whether you think you can or think you can't, you're right.*
> – Henry Ford

illness, sometimes even making the difference in whether they live or die. This can be seen with heart illness, where the right eating habits, appropriate exercise, and stress management can save your heart and your life. On the other hand, denying the existence of your illness and refusing to make changes that are necessary for health can lead you toward life-threatening decisions.

Many psychologists believe that how you think greatly affects what you do and how you feel. They believe that changing your thoughts will cause you to act and feel differently. Some psychologists also go on to say that changing how you act may change how you think and feel.

Brain Chemistry and Attitude

There are two distinct approaches you can use to help your attitude and related brain chemistry. The first approach is learning how to judge whether or not your thoughts are healthy and logical. Unhealthy thoughts can have an enormous effect on you mood, accompanying attitudes, and your brain chemistry. Learning how to look at your thoughts realistically can help you change unhealthy thought patterns. Research has shown, through blood flow changes measured by sophisticated Positron Emission Tomography (PET) scans, that just talking through a bad attitude with someone else can have a healthy effect on your brain chemistry.

> *The last of the human freedoms is to choose one's attitude.*
>
> – Victor Frankl

A second way to help your attitude is the use of proper medication. Much has been written about brain chemistry and how antidepressant medications can change how a person feels about himself or herself by changing thoughts and mood. Today, medication is available to help make a pessimistic person think like an optimist! Well, almost!

Medication may give a person enough energy to cope with the many life challenges that life-changing illness presents. You may be unable to take the active steps that may help benefit your mood, such as reading or exercise. For example, when you are feeling "down in the dumps," it may be very hard to get moving to take a walk or read a novel, even though you know intellectually that either activity might help you feel better. If medication helps your mood, which in turn aids in improving your thoughts, then you may then be able to convince yourself that taking a walk or reading a good novel might indeed help you feel better.

How Medication Can Promote a Healthy Attitude

Many people do not want to take medication to help with feelings of depression or anxiety. You may be one of those people. If so, you are not alone. However, we encourage you to talk to your doctor if you know your mood is affecting your lifestyle. If someone is telling you that you are not yourself, listen to him or her. Friends can be good mirrors.

Although friends can be good mirrors, you and your physician need to determine whether your illness, other medications you are taking, or reaction to your illness are causing your depressed or anxious feelings. Sometimes your illness directly affects your mood. Thyroid disease is a good example. When your thyroid blood level is too high, you tend to feel anxious, nervous and jittery no matter how hard you try to hold onto peaceful and calm thoughts. If your thyroid blood level is too low, you may feel tired, lethargic, and depressed no matter how many walks you take to boost your mood.

> *In the face of uncertainty, there is nothing wrong with hope.*
>
> – Bernie S. Seigel, M.D.

The second reason for your depression or anxiety involves the medications used to treat your illness, some of which may cause unpleasant side effects. If a medication has been prescribed, you probably need the medication or a substitute for it. It is important not to stop any medication without your physician's approval, even if you suspect it of affecting your mood. There may be a simple solution to your unpleasant feelings if you communicate them to your prescribing physician.

The third reason for your mood change may be reaction to your illness. Coping and reacting to your illness can bring out emotions that nobody likes. They are a realistic part of the adjustment to life-changing illness. If these emotions are keeping you from doing activities you used to enjoy, don't hesitate to talk to your physician. Your physician is an important ally to help sort out why you feel the way you do.

If medication is prescribed, it is important to take the medication exactly as your physician recommends. If you experience unpleasant side effects, call your physician or nurse. Often side effects go away or can be controlled easily after a limited unpleasant adjustment period.

If you and your physician determine that a medication may help you, we encourage you to try it. Medication can be very effective, especially when combined with counseling to help you analyze your thinking patterns. We believe the advice of Tipper Gore, Mental Health Policy Advisor to President Clinton, is succinct:

> When you get to this point of being seriously depressed…you can't just will your way out of that or pray your way out of that or pull yourself up by the bootstraps out of that. You really have to go and get help. (Psychology Today, June 2000, "Our Mental Health Awards" p. 52.)

Attitudes, Actions, and Beliefs

Let's return now to the subject of attitude. After you have partnered with your medical doctor to determine if medication is appropriate, it is time to begin to look at how you can help yourself with a healthy attitude. With or without medication, a look at your attitudes and beliefs can be an important step toward feeling better.

> *When one door of happiness closes, another opens; but often we look so long at the closed door that we do not see the one which has opened for us.*
>
> — Helen Keller

Attitudes and actions are important because those of us with life-changing illness more than everyone else need to be taking healthy actions. For example, if you have had a heart attack, your doctor may have recommended that you stop smoking or lose weight. These life changes are very hard to make, as you know if you have tried to stop smoking or lose weight. If you add attitudes that say "I can never do this" or "Why should I change, I am not going to live long anyway," your probability of changing those lifestyle habits decreases dramatically.

If your attitude is "I will do this change one day at a time and a slip up is just that, a slip up," you are much more likely to accomplish and maintain healthy changes. Your attitude (thought) change can help you become successful in your actions. How different do you think you might feel if you view each day as *mostly a success* instead of totally a failure because of one cookie you ate or one cigarette you smoked?

There are specific thinking patterns that have been found to contribute to negative or positive attitudes. We will define these patterns and help you learn to recognize them. If different thinking patterns are something that you believe might improve your lifestyle, then study these ideas that experts think can help you attain a healthy attitude. Belief systems do affect your attitude. It has been proven that your attitude actually affects your body's chemistry and how your brain functions. Your attitude can make a powerful difference in being able to cope with the adjustments in life that you must constantly be making with your life-changing illness.

Recognizing Beliefs That Strangle a Healthy Attitude

Cognitive-behavioral psychologists have developed a list of negative, unhealthy, unrealistic thoughts that people commonly practice. These are thoughts everyone has at times that can keep him or her from seeing a more realistic world or making healthy lifestyle changes.

> *Sometimes you just need to look reality in the eye and deny it.*
>
> – Garrison Keillor

We want to offer a word of caution. Because we are comparing attitudes you may have with attitudes people in general have about life, you may react by saying to yourself, "But that is true, it is that way in my life." You might be saying, "But I feel bad because I am sick! How dare anyone say I am depressed!" We understand your reaction because we have similar thoughts. Much of your sadness, anxiousness, negative thoughts and beliefs are valid because they are related to adapting to your illness. We do not deny that. However, if you take a second look at your situation, you will often find that your thought about your situation is not a perfectly correct statement. We will discuss how to determine the difference a little later. The important thing is to remember that your thoughts and beliefs color your reaction to events. The reaction (feelings and actions) that follows those thoughts and beliefs can make the difference in how you live out your life with a life-changing illness.

A negative attitude can distort your view of your health situation and strangle you from positive thinking. Take a moment to think about a distorted picture on your television set. Unless a message comes on the screen telling you that the problem is not in your set, you know that a picture signal was transmitted from the television station. The picture is still there. However, you also know that something has changed how the picture looks to you, making it difficult for you to interpret that picture accurately. In much the same way, your negative attitude can distort the reality of your illness. Things may be bad, but not as bad as they look through your attitude-influenced view, which strangles you from thinking positively.

The following is a list of thoughts that produce negative thinking that can color or distort your thoughts and reactions. You may find yourself guilty of falling into one or more of these thought patterns. We certainly do!

Strangling Patterns of Thinking

- **Generalizing excessively.** You project one negative event into a trend or epidemic of problems.

- **Exaggerating or minimizing a situation.** You make "mountains out of mole hills" or just the opposite, deny the seriousness of a situation.

- **Seeing everything in black and white.** Things look absolute. There is no middle ground.

- **Dwelling on the negatives or ignoring the positives.** You might be overly pessimistic.

- **Inaccurate reasoning.** You may let your feelings totally take over your thinking. Reasoning requires both thinking and feeling.

- **Thinking in *shoulds, woulds, coulds*.** You criticize yourself or other people for what should, could, or would have been done.

- **Labeling.** You may call yourself or other people unflattering names.

- **Playing the blame game with yourself and others.** You might burn up energy assigning blame instead of working on solutions.

- **Worrying excessively.** No explanation needed here.

- **Reading minds.** You may reach conclusions by thinking you know what other people are thinking or what they will do before they happen.

- **Perfection.** You may feel unworthy if you are anything less than perfect.

- **Fortune telling.** Being sure of what will happen in the future, especially the negative.

Patients have a wide range of views of illness, some of which are positive while others are negative. For instance, your experience with illness can be viewed as a challenge, puzzle, or problem to solve, presenting you a life situation that consists of multiple tasks that must be mastered. On the other hand, you may see illness as an enemy that needs to be fought, like an invasion of harmful forces that entered your life and body. (Just the word enemy may conger up a drain on your energy.)

You might see illness as a punishment, sign of weakness, or as a lost opportunity, being delivered justly or unjustly because of your lack of perfection. As an alternative, you may see your illness as a relief that allows you to escape from your typical life stresses or as a strategy you may use in trying to get more attention from your family and friends. Often illness causes irreparable loss; your dreams may be much harder to reach. Finally, illness may also be an opportunity to become a person who looks at life through a new set of glasses. You may use your illness for growth and development.

These reactions to illness can contribute to healthy feelings and behaviors. Other reactions are likely to contribute to negative feelings and behaviors. Some of these views about illness may lead to either positive or negative feelings and positive or negative behaviors depending on how your previous experiences have taught you to react.

For example, if you view your illness as a relief from your typical life stresses, you can react to that belief in a couple of ways. One way would be for you to sit back and play the sick role. You might need to stop working because of your illness. Not working may be important, as you can no longer physically handle the strain or stress your body has from that employment. However, if that causes you to sit at home and do nothing and allow others to wait on you unnecessarily, then seeing your illness as a relief is not healthy for you or for your relationships with others. A second reaction to seeing your illness as a relief could be to see what positive changes you can make in those life stresses to make life better for you and your family. You may now have the time available to spend more time with loved ones. You may still not be able to work, but you can use your illness and attitude as an opportunity for change to a healthier life.

> *Experience is not what happens to a man. It is what a man does with what happens to him.*
>
> – Aldous Huxley

You may relate to these views of illness. You may feel differently about your illness depending what day it is. We certainly have good days and bad days. We sometimes feel a tremendous loss and grief from our illness. Only occasionally can we see our illness as an opportunity.

Carol's father had to take disability from his job as an electrical engineer due to his heart problems. When asked what he thought about not being able to work, he told about a dream. In the dream he was asked to complete a project at work. In the dream, he would get a big smile on his face, put his feet up on his desk, and say, "I'm retired!" The word "retired" was his way of reframing his disability into a benefit. Taking early retirement was a positive change for him. We are sure that he would have preferred not to have heart disease, but if he had to be ill, then he at least could see disability and retirement as a relief.

Doug did not want to take disability from his employment as a partner in an international consulting firm, but he eventually realized that it was a necessary step to take. He still hesitates occasionally when someone asks him what he "does for a living." He is too young to say "retired" without getting a strange look or follow-up question. He has rehearsed many times how to explain his situation in a short sentence. However, he does try to look at his nonworking situation as an opportunity. Although he is not able to continue his chosen career, he is able to spend time volunteering and writing. His illness slows him down significantly, which has forced him to focus more than ever before on deciding what is important and being more proactive in planning where he spends his energy.

Methods to Analyze Attitude

Before you become too hard on yourself, remember that when your illness or other events give you stress, most people naturally experience the kinds of thought distortions listed in the "Strangling Patterns of Thinking" earlier in this chapter. Nonetheless, these thoughts are dangerous and can cause you further stress. Often these thoughts are unrealistic or only partially realistic. Therefore, you need to learn techniques to discriminate between your healthy and true thoughts and your stress-producing distorted thinking.

In terms of the think-feel-do cycle discussed earlier, you may see that you are cycling downward. Each cycle can make you feel worse, act worse, and then think badly of yourself. Taking time to put your finger on the thoughts that are preventing you from improving your attitude is very important. We will outline one of these methods to help you analyze your thoughts. A blank copy of this worksheet is available at www.patientpress.com and may be copied for your personal non-commercial use.

One effective method for analyzing your attitude uses journaling to sort out what is going on inside your brain. We developed the following worksheet based on cognitive behavioral theory for assessing what is happening. For people who already keep a journal or like to write, using this tool will be fairly easy. However, if the closest you get to writing is putting appointments in your calendar, this method may be more of a challenge. If you are one of the second type of people, try writing about your situation or an event once a day in your daily calendar or other convenient space.

The thought review sheet is an example of how you can analyze and keep track of your thoughts about what is happening inside your brain.

Thought Review Worksheet

1. Describe the event, situation or action.

2. How I felt before, during and after the event, situation, or action.

3. My thoughts, both negative and positive, about the above. (Rate each thought on a scale of 0 to 10, with 10 being the strongest belief at the time.)

4. What actions happened because of my thoughts?

5. Check the "Strangling Patterns of Thinking" list. Which of the above thoughts match one of the patterns.

6. If necessary, can I change this thought distortion so that it is more accurate?

7. How might that change how I would feel and what I would do if the event were to occur again?

This process becomes easier after you do several of the thought journals. You may want to try doing two or three of them with a trusted family member, friend, mentor, pastor or counselor who can help you sort out your situation. Pick someone from whom you can accept honest feedback. After writing several, you will soon be able to take a calendar out at the end of the day, do this exercise in brief, in your head, and then write down the action or event and the thought distortion involved and rate how strongly you believe it to be. You can use other experiences to prove to yourself the reality of the thinking distortion pattern. In time and with the other experiences, you will hopefully see your belief in the distortion become less and less.

The following Thought Review Worksheet is based on an example from Carol's life.

Thought Review Worksheet

1. Describe the event, situation, or action.

When I was attending a conference out-of-town, I had chest pain and shortness of breath during a fire alarm. I had to be carried out by my husband and a man who was attending the same conference.

2. How I felt before, during and after the event, situation, or action.

embarrassment, fear of dying, out of control, anger at the situation I have to live with

3. My thoughts, both negative and positive, about the above. (Rate each thought on a scale of 0 to 10, with 10 being the strongest beliefs at the time.)

#1 I was dying. *Rate as 4*

#2 I will look silly to my fellow classmates who were sure to see me. *Rate as 4*

#3 I can't count on my health and should never travel away from my doctors. *Rate as 10*

#4 I will never be well enough to do the things I want to do. *Rate as 9*

4. What actions happened because of my thoughts?

#1 I allowed the paramedics to check me even though my symptoms had passed.

#2 I was so embarrassed that I closed my eyes so as not to look at them at the door during the alarm and so as to relax. I talked a lot about my health condition when I went back to the seminar so the people would not think I was making a big deal about nothing.

#3 Before my next trip I had my doctor write a detailed medical history and more forcefully requested to be on the first floor at the next hotel I stayed in.

#4 I was angry for a while and I talked it through with Doug and friends to see the reality of the situation.

5. Check the "Strangling Patterns of Thinking" list. Which above thoughts match one of the patterns.

Inaccurate reasoning (note my use of Never), generalizing excessively (will never be able to do), fortune telling (about my future abilities), labeling (I look silly)

6. If necessary, can I change this thought distortion so that it is more accurate?

(#1) I may be dying, but most likely this is a symptom of my heart disease combined with extra activity, it will pass when I rest. (#2) My fellow classmates are medical people and will understand the precautions of being carried and the paramedics. #3 Slow down my thought process, one step at a time, I cannot possibly know this answer today. (#4) Know that I have had this thought before and it has been incorrect and it may also be incorrect now, so take a deep breath and take a "wait and see" attitude for now.

7. **How might that change how you would feel and what you would do if the event were to occur again?**

My fears would greatly decrease and I would know not to make hasty decisions about the future which would allow me to put my energy on relaxing for health and toward calming down in my head (thoughts that could not help at that moment.)

We now suggest that you take out a sheet of paper and try the exercise for yourself. Later in this chapter we will talk about other types of journaling. Verbalizing your thoughts either written on paper or to another empathetic person is very helpful in clearing out your brain cobwebs which are full of a strangling attitudes and painful emotions.

Attitude Tapes

You may have heard people refer to the thoughts or messages that play over and over in their heads from earlier life experiences as "old tapes." Everyone has tapes from earlier events, even from childhood. These can either poison or fertilize reactions to events surrounding life-changing illness. Your core beliefs have been unconsciously learned from events and circumstances over an entire lifetime. Many of these circumstances occurred in early childhood. Seeing an event through a child's eyes does not give a balanced view of the world. Because children do not have a full range of life experiences, they often find it impossible to see an event in proper perspective. Even so, these events early in life can color attitudes about yourself and others and about your reaction to events many years later.

For example, if as a child you received an inoculation against disease every time you went to the doctor's office, you may have inferred that going to a doctor is painful and even scary. You had no reference to see that your doctor had long-term benefit for your health. Today's thoughts of fear about going to the doctor may be based on a childhood tape that you learned many years ago that says, "You will receive pain when you go to the doctor." You may not even know such a tape is playing; you just know that you feel anxious or scared when you go to the doctor's office.

Evaluating these attitudes or "tapes" is worth the time and effort that the evaluation takes. You can make a new recording in your head to replace the old tape. "Doctors have knowledge that may help my life-changing illness" is a much healthier thought. Thinking and beginning to believe that will reduce the stress that your childhood-based fears provoke. Believing that going to your doctor may help you, may prompt you to call the doctor rather than avoiding making the call. Thus, you may get help for a problem before it becomes a crisis.

Although the process of answering the questions on the worksheet or solving the goose riddle may not be easy, it is worth your time and energy. If your head is full of old tapes that are making your life harder, then questioning those tapes and erasing the negative ones can benefit your life. If you can visualize yourself outside of the bottle where you can stretch your goose wings, your life can be less restricted by illness. Life with life-changing illness has enough challenges without giving yourself extra ones produced by believing in old false tapes or putting yourself into a bottle like the goose.

Developing a Stress-Hardy Attitude

If you could take a safe, simple pill that would make you invulnerable to stress, you would take it in a minute and thus be free of the "side effects" of stress. But there is no such pill! To control stress in your life you must take control of your life. There is no passive solution. However, you can integrate some attitude characteristics into your life.

Dr. Suzanne Kobasa, while testing individuals in the workplace, found that people with certain characteristics were more "stress-hardy." Workers with stress-hardy characteristics showed decreased incidence of illness and decreased absenteeism from work. There were three associated personality characteristics, which Dr. Kobasa called the three Cs: *control*, *challenge*, and *commitment*.

The Mind/Body Medical Institute's Ann Webster believes from her clinical experience that there is a fourth C, *closeness*. If you feel connected to other people who are supportive, you may be more stress-hardy. The following chart compares stress-producing thoughts and stress-hardy thoughts.

Four Cs of the Stress-Hardy Person

Characteristic	Stress-Producing Belief	Stress-Hardy Belief
Control	I am out of control or I have no control over events in my life.	I can control life by making good choices and influencing events around me.
Challenge	I am incapable of successfully handling this challenge.	I view this challenge as a new opportunity for growth.
Commitment	I do not want to be involved.	I am interested in being involved in activities and people around me.
Closeness	I feel isolated, alone, and unsupported.	I have friends who support and care about me.

Do you recognize yourself in any of the stress-producing thinking patterns in the second column above? If you do, take time to study them. See how you can change your attitude and approach to life both in thought and action. Try one of the stress-hardy beliefs from column three for a day. You could even use it as a statement during your mini relaxation exercises. See if thinking one of these beliefs can make any difference in how you think, feel, and act.

The four Cs that can help people cope with general stress also can help those of us with stress as a result of our illness.

Writing to Clear Out Your Brain's Cobwebs

Writing is another technique to help you improve your attitude. People have been writing journals, diaries and pillow books for centuries. Many young girls have had one of those little "locking" diaries in which they told of their hopes and dreams, loves and sorrows. Anne Frank's diary of her teenage experience during the holocaust is required reading for many youth.

Many have found that writing about their troubles, fears, losses, and anger gives perspective on their circumstances and solace that they may have been missing. Some people even write about past painful and traumatic events, and then discover that they can finally put the past behind them. Psychologist James W. Pennebaker and colleagues, psychologist Janice K. Kiecolt-Glaser and her husband immunologist Ronald Glaser, completed groundbreaking research in the early 1990s. Their research showed that writing about your deepest, most overwhelming, and traumatic experiences and emotions, for as little as 20 minutes a day for four days, can heighten your immune function when compared with people who wrote about superficial topics. Their research showed that this immune function effect continued for six weeks. Not surprisingly the students who wrote about traumatic experiences also visited the college health center less often. (James W. Pennebaker, Ph.D., *Opening Up: The Healing Power of Expressing Emotions,* New York: Guilford Press, 1997, pp. 30-37.) If four days of journaling can be so powerful for those student/research subjects, imagine what daily writing may be able to do for you!

A recent study reported in *The Journal of the American Medical Association* (JAMA) found that writing about emotionally traumatic experiences can benefit patients' health by reducing physical symptoms in patients with asthma and rheumatoid arthritis. These improvements were measured with tests and went beyond expected improvements from traditional standard care. The improvements continued for four months. Writing helps people with chronic symptoms without need for more medication and without negative side effects. (*The Journal of the American Medical Association* (JAMA), 1999, 281:1304-1309, Joshua M. Smyth, Ph.D.; Arthur A. Stone, Ph.D.; Adam Hurewitz, M.D.; Alan Kaell, M.D., "Effects of Writing About Stressful Experiences on Symptom Reduction in Patients With Asthma or Rheumatoid Arthritis: A Randomized Trial".)

Even with these very convincing recommendations, writing is a chore for many people. You may feel like nothing you write is any good or you may remember what your teachers criticized about your school papers. Sometimes even your childhood penmanship grades makes putting pen to the paper a task that reminds you of a difficult teacher who ridiculed your Ps or Q. The good news is that the writing that clears out your brain's cobwebs does not have anything to do with the writing assignments you were given as a child. There are few, if any, rules!

Even though journaling is different from the writing you may remember from school, it does take some tricks to get started if you are one of those people who remember more criticism than compliments about writing. Here is a list of *dos and don'ts* for getting started.

1. Find a place that is as quiet and as far away from disturbances as possible.

2. Go buy yourself a pen and notebook that you like and that feel comfortable in your hands. It may be helpful to buy a set of multicolored pens so you can choose a color that relates to your mood of the day.

3. If you are a computer user, using the word processor can be a tool to help you express your thoughts.

4. Find a safe spot to store your journal so that what you write is for your eyes only. With a computer, that may mean finding a password that can protect your words from other eyes.

Now you are ready for the next step, putting your fingers to the keyboard or your pen to the paper. Here is a list to get your words flowing.

1. Begin with a moment or two of silence to allow your mind to settle and the thoughts you want to write about to form. Take a few deep breaths or do a mini relaxation.

2. When you start to write, do so as fast as your can. Do not restrict or censure yourself, just keep the pen moving.

3. Do not worry about correcting your words. Foul words, misspelled words, poor handwriting and bad grammar are permitted here.

4. Be absolutely honest with yourself and your piece of paper.

5. Allow balance in what you write about. Although the research we mentioned earlier in this section used traumatic writing, not all of your writing needs to be about terrible thoughts and experiences. Take time to write about the present moment as you are experiencing it. Write about experiences that you enjoy such as your favorite vacation, a special relative, or a joyful moment in a child's life that you witness.

Sometimes a structure within which to write is needed to get the pen moving. In fact, Carol first began journaling regularly when she learned some specific exercises to use to get her pen in motion. Structure provides a margin of comfort for those new or uncomfortable with the journal process. Pacing and containment allow you to know this is only for a certain amount of time. Here are some easy starters.

- **Five minute sprints.** Set a timer and just start writing, knowing that in five minutes you can stop.

- **Lists.** Start with a list of 100 places you would like to visit or your 100 favorite people. This is a "keep the pen moving exercise." Do not worry about writing the same thing more than once. That happens when you are tapping your unconscious thoughts. Look at the repeats when you are done; are there any surprises or themes that stand out for you?

- **Unsent letters.** Write all of those thoughts that you can't say out loud or that you think of after your discussion with the person. This is also helpful when you can no longer talk with the person such as after death or divorce. Go for it, no holding back because no one else will ever see these words.

- **Character sketch.** Describe a person you know or have known. They may be real or fictional. You may also use this to describe yourself or even a part of your personality.

- **Alphapoems.** Write the letters of the alphabet down the side of a piece of paper. Pick a topic such as how it feels to hurt all the time. Now fill in each letter with a line related to the topic. The only rule is that the first word starts with the letter on that line of the paper. See the example of this starter on the following page.

Resources are available to help you start the writing process. Kathleen Adams of The Center for Journal Therapy has written several books on this topic. They include *Journal to the Self: Twenty-two Paths To Personal Growth, The Way of the Journal* and *The Write to Wellness: A Workbook for Healing and Change*. Her resources are available at http://www.journaltherapy.com. The subject of the April, 2000 issue of the e-zine Soulful Living.com (http://www.soulfulliving.com/aprilfeatures.htm) is "Writing for Reflection and Intention." This e-zine includes many resources for journaling. A third resource is Sue Meyn's site http://www.journalmagic.com. She includes topics and suggestions to help with journal writing and will send you a weekly topic to journal about. She also offers a tool for sale called "Journal Cards," which can be found on her Internet site.

Writing can be fun, it can be healthy, it can improve your physical symptoms, it can strengthen your immune system, and it can improve your thoughts and attitudes. Writing gives you a new view of life and some perspective on your feelings. So write for health, it may be your doctor's next prescription.

An Alphapoem by Carol:
When I Cannot Sleep I Feel…

Awful.

Bound up inside my covers.

Can't can't can't sleep!

Don't want to think

Elephant size thoughts.

Fighting sleepiness.

Going to get up.

Haunting things I did.

Illness becomes larger.

Joking this is not. Wish I could float like a…

Kite.

Lemonade might refresh my tired body.

Make up sheep to count.

Nobody knows or cares that I can not sleep because they ARE sleeping.

Only someone NOT sleeping understands.

Please, please, God, let me sleep.

Quaint rocker might soothe my angry thoughts.

Rock and rock to childlike lullabies of innocence.

Simple thoughts please envelop me.

Tired, I am so tired, I am so very tired….

Underneath my skin, my frustrations of sleepless thoughts show.

Very new.

What can I do?

Xerox a copy of me sleeping,

You would know then,

Zero sleep is no fun!

Humor for Health

A familiar Biblical passage (Proverb 17:22) says, "A cheerful heart is good medicine." Another popular adage says, "Laughter is good medicine." Research shows that a belly laugh does wonders for releasing endorphins, those "feel good" pain-relieving juices that your body produces. Even something as minor as just changing your facial expression to a smile can change your body chemistry and your thoughts.

The following are benefits of therapeutic humor:

- Reduces stress

- Boosts immunity

- Relieves pain

- Decreases anxiety

- Stabilizes mood

- Rests the brain

- Enhances communication

- Inspires creativity

- Maintains hope

- Bolsters morale

(From Peggy Wooten's Web site, www.jesthealth.com/bene.html.)

Try to smile for a minute, even if you do not feel like smiling. What thoughts and feelings do you have? Next make a frown. What thoughts and feelings come to mind when you frown? Now, put on the smile again and try to think a pessimistic thought—like "I will never get my work done today." The thought doesn't match your face, does it? You can think of your smile as a button to activate your neurohormones and neurotransmitters,

> *The human race has one really effective weapon, and that is laughter.*
>
> – Mark Twain

your natural "feel good" medicine. Putting on a happy face can be good medicine; doing so will probably make you feel at least a little better.

Humor is powerful. However, there is a big "but" to consider when talking about humor in connection with illness. Being sick isn't usually very funny. Inappropriate humor from the wrong person can make you feel irritated and sometimes downright angry. There are several types of unhealthy humor.

- **Hostile humor.** If the joker uses jokes or other humorous statements to release hostile, cynical emotions, which make you feel embarrassed, humiliated, or resentful of that person, then that isn't healthy humor. No one feels better after hearing a sarcastic comment hurled toward someone.

- **Untimely or inappropriate humor.** Sometimes humor used to "cheer you up" is not well received. This humor communicates that the giver may not see or understand the seriousness of the situation, may feel uncomfortable talking about your situation seriously, or may be trying to "fix" your mood. It is OK for you to just need to know that your friend sees your emotional and physical pain and is comfortable with sitting with you and listening.

We remember a painful example of untimely humor, when a friend visited us as we waited for Carol to go into cardiac pacemaker surgery. The friend, apparently trying to be uplifting, was "yucking it up" with jokes and comments that were less than soothing during an anxious wait for surgery. In that situation, simply being with us and letting us take the lead with the conversation would have been more consoling.

In situations where the humor giver and receiver know and understand one another, humor can be a wonderful break from the serious, sad or painful sides of illness. The "apple juice or urine?" jokes have probably been overused but they can change a mood, even if just for the moment. Laughing at yourself or exaggerating a situation can help you feel better by changing your perspective.

Try to find a way to purposefully give yourself a daily dose of humor.

- **Read.** Read a book by a humorous author such as Erma Bombeck and Loretta LaRouche.

- **Scrapbook.** Make a scrapbook with cut out cartoons. Carol has never forgotten one of a man looking at his IV glucose bag saying with a look of horror, "There is a fly in my glucose!"

- **Odd twists.** When you see a funny twist or a play on words, remember it and use it. More often than Carol wishes to hear, Doug says, "Wow I could have had an IV, a play on an old commercial for V-8 juice. Carol called herself "The Bionic Woman," when she received her first cardiac pacemaker in 1979, inspired by the 1970s television series.

- **Movies.** Watch a funny movie or television show. The oldies that you can get on videotape, like Charlie Chaplin, "The Three Stooges," and "I Love Lucy," are some of the best. When you watch a funny movie, find a friend to watch it with you. A friend's laugh can trigger you to laugh also.

- **Bulletin board.** Make a bulletin board at your home, office or hospital room with funny bumper stickers, pictures or signs.

In short, give yourself opportunities to smile and laugh. It is guaranteed to give you a momentary change of attitude. With enough opportunities humor may even help you feel better.

Summary

Attitude matters!

This chapter has reminded you how important your attitude is to your overall well-being. More importantly, you have the power to reshape and change your attitude toward almost everything, especially your illness and the extent to which it defines you. This chapter has offered you numerous suggestions for analyzing your attitudes and reshaping them to develop a stress-hardy attitude. You have also been reminded of the power of writing, through journaling, and the power of humor.

Maintaining a "healthy" attitude, when your body isn't so healthy, is no easy task. That is one reason it is important to become skilled at understanding and meeting your personal needs, and not feel guilty about it. In the next chapter, "Nurturing Yourself," you will learn some of the keys to taking care of those needs.

Hope is a risk that must be run.

– George Bernanos

TEN

NURTURING YOURSELF

Self-nurture is not about being selfish.
It is about self-care.

– Alica D. Domar, Ph.D.

*M*ost of this book has been focused on you, offering tools to help you cope with your life-changing illness. We have offered suggestions to help you live your life better within the context of your life-changing illness. We have offered these suggestions because we believe they will be helpful to you, based on our own experience as patients.

You might be feeling that we are telling you to take these prescriptions for living because "it's good for you." Instead, we want you to believe that you deserve to be good to yourself just because you are a unique and special person. So this chapter is about being good to yourself in ways that are unique to you.

Despite the feelings of guilt or selfishness that most people have, there is at least some of the time when we need to do something for ourselves. It is good to take care of yourself, to have fun, and to find pleasure. To find out what is nurturing for you, there are several questions you need to ask.

- What do I like to do?

- What am I good at doing?

- What brings me comfort?

- How am I energized?

- How do I as a unique individual need to be cared for?

After you have answered these questions, you will more easily know when to say "yes" to yourself without someone else telling you what you should do. Only you know yourself. You may have a life-changing illness, feel as if you *are* an illness, and be convinced you are unable to do anything more, but you are much more than an illness. We believe that being good to yourself is also beneficial to your health. By beginning to know yourself better, we hope you will be more able to nurture yourself.

In this chapter, we will focus on who you are and what you need so that you can take care of yourself. Some of the topics we will look at include the following:

- The Time Pie of Your Life

- Using Your Senses to Care for and Comfort Yourself

  - Sound

- Sight

- Smell

- Touch

• Knowing Your Talents and Gifts

• Reaching Out to Others to Nurture Yourself

• Connecting with Others and Communicating Your Special Needs

• Summary

The Time Pie of Your Life

Most people tend to go through life living and doing what they are "supposed to do." Doing the right thing might mean working hard at your job. It may mean being the best parent or approaching parenting the way your neighbors or your parents expect you to do. Perhaps it means saying "yes" once or twice or even three times too many to this or that committee assignment or project. You may believe family needs should always come before your own need. (Oops, there is that "should" word we talked about in Chapter Nine, "Realigning Your Attitude," not to mention the code word for generalizing excessively, "always.") The word "no" never enters your mind or you feel like you will have a large guilt attack if you do say "no."

To choose time is to save time.

— Francis Bacom

Sometimes you can get lost in the world of "supposed to do's." We have had this happen to us often. For example, we've attended work-related social events that weren't really important only because we felt obligated to attend. Participating in these drained our energy, making it harder to do things we truly valued, like getting together with friends. Many times we have said "yes" when we should have said "no." Sometimes we say "yes" to an activity that we don't even like to do! Why? Maybe it is because we feel obligated. Maybe we like the person who is asking us to do something. Maybe we think it will make us feel better about ourselves. When we say "yes" to something we don't really want to do, the activity takes a toll on our health. We may get tired, irritable or compromise our health, which is not the greatest to begin with.

When Carol was a co-chair of the Nurture & Care Committee at our church, she would often tell volunteers, "You cannot help someone else if you are not taking care of yourself. Don't say yes if this is one too many for you now, and don't feel guilty." She knew this from experience, often having realized it after she had said "yes" one too many times. If Carol volunteered for too many activities at her son's elementary school, she could not be an effective mother to him when he came home at the end of the school day.

In today's culture, the times that someone offers you an opportunity to nurture yourself and helps you avoid your guilt trip after saying "no" are very few. Thus, each person must learn to say "no" especially when "no" means saying "yes" to taking care of him- or herself. No one else can do this.

Harvard Medical School's Mind/Body Medical Institute's Dr. Ann Webster uses a time pie to help her clients with AIDS and cancer. Her clients are in symptom reduction groups. This exercise helps them to realize just how much or how little time they allocate for themselves during any given day or week.

Most of us are unaware of how little time we allow in any given day for nurturing ourselves. What would your 24-hour time pie look like? Putting a visual time pie down on paper is a graphic way to see what percentage of the day you are doing something for you. Consider that in a 24-hour day, you probably spend eight hours sleeping, maybe more if you need a rest period during the day. Consider how much time you spend at your job, which could be another eight or more hours a day if you work full time. After you consider travel time, medical appointments, cooking, grocery shopping, maintaining your house and yard, and keeping up with children's activities, you can see pretty quickly that unless you carve out specific slices of time for yourself, the time for you will not happen.

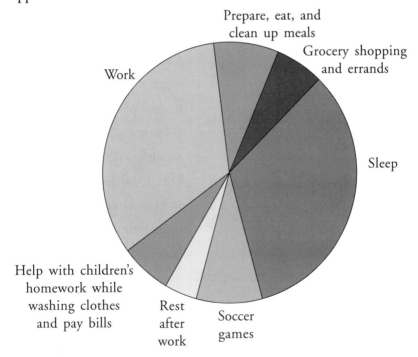

Like other people with life-changing illness, you may find it especially difficult to carve out time for yourself. In addition to the many ways life calls everyone to duty, you also must take out time to rest, go to the doctor, or due to lengthy regimens to regain or keep what strength you have. For some people, even dressing can be a daunting task. By the time you are ready for the day, you are too tired to think about self-care. Yet research tells you that taking time to take care of yourself is exactly what you need. From the mind/body connection, it has been shown that self-care increases the good secretions like pleasure-causing endorphins, mood stabilizers like seratonin, and immune-strengthening hormones. At the conclusion of this chapter, go back to your own time pie and find a place to add on at least one or two nurturing activities each day.

Using Your Senses to Care for and Comfort Yourself

All living things, including human beings, need nourishment in their lives. Imagine a common houseplant in your home, a beautiful, lush, flowering plant. You may be thinking something like, "Me, have a plant! Plants wilt if I even look at them in the store, much less if I bring one home. Dead within the week!" Without nurture and a skilled green thumb, every green plant brought home will most certainly wither and die very quickly. With an adequate dose of water in a timely fashion, a spoonful of the right fertilizer, and a window with some sun, almost every plant can flourish. Even if bugs or disease come in contact with the plant, a well-nurtured plant stands a much better chance of surviving.

> *The kiss of sun for pardon,*
> *The song of the birds for mirth —*
> *One is nearer God's Heart*
> *in a garden*
> *Than anywhere else on earth.*
>
> – Dorothy Gurney

Just as care and the right ingredients produce a happy plant, you can create a healthier and happier self with special care. Even with life-changing illness there are things you can do to be good to both your mind and your body.

Do you nurture yourself to keep your mind, body, and spirit happy? Do you allow yourself the essential time and effort that must be taken for self-nurture? If not, you are far from alone. Finding time for yourself is very difficult. Allowing your senses to be actively sensing may take some assertive behavior. For example, if you are a parent of young children, you may need to shut a door for a period of time when they are safe with someone else. If you are at home most of the time living with a spouse or roommate, you may need to say, "I need some time alone to go for a walk every day and to eat on a regular schedule in order to take care of my body. So please understand that when I take this time; it is about caring for me, not a negative reaction toward you."

The following are descriptive lists of ways to nurture your senses. When you find several ways that help you, be persistent about finding time to take advantage of these nurturing activities.

Sound

Music has a powerful effect on your emotional and physical state through your sense of hearing. From ancient times until today people have been using music for many purposes. Examples include:

- Soothing and healing (kings had court minstrels)

- Enhancing romance (couples label a song "our song")

- Proclaiming victory (such as the "Star Spangled Banner" or the use of Scottish Bagpipes)

We recommend that you try to find what music and sound works best to make you feel better. To nurture your sense of hearing, the first step you must take is to become aware of whether you like to have noise of any kind or tend to prefer silence. You may or may not like noise. For example, in our family, Carol prefers silence to "noises" like talk radio and televised sports. On the other hand, Doug often appreciates the distraction of just those things! He doesn't consider it distraction. He enjoys hearing the banter, finding out the many sides of a breaking story or sports event. The talking keeps his mind from dwelling on negative thoughts. We know a mother of twins who occasionally wore a radio headset to get some relief from the constant noise of two loud young children.

> *The hills are alive with the sound of music.*
>
> – Oscar Hammerstein

Scientists have found that music helps trigger the release of endorphins, chemicals that relieve pain and induce a state of euphoria. Researchers have found that music affects your mind. Their research has shown how music may help you relax, heal, and may increase your concentration for learning.

Your body can become "entrained" to music, meaning that your heart beat and breathing slow down or speed up in direct response to various beats. For an application of this think about your reaction to a suspense-thriller movie. Listen to the music the next time. The music is expertly dubbed into the picture to "aid" or "enhance" your frightened response. Try to remain aloof from that fear reaction. You will likely find it will be very difficult to filter out your reaction to the music. Just as fear can be musically tuned into you, a state of relaxation for your body can be tuned with music.

Begin your search to find out what sounds nourish you by selectively removing certain sounds for a time. Does it cause you to feel like something is missing or does it give you what Carol calls that "aahhhhh" feeling that she gets when Doug turns off his talk radio?

After you know some of what you do and don't like within your world, think about adding different new sounds. Do the sounds of the ocean soothe you when you're on vacation? Do you like to hear the birds when you have the windows open in the spring? Do you enjoy hearing the rain on your roof on a rainy afternoon? One or all of these sounds may soothe you. If you do not have access to the real thing, a compact diskplayer can almost duplicate the sound in your home. Try one out and see if it gives you a nourishing atmosphere. Try out music with some of the nifty headsets they have at music stores or check out music on an Internet site such as Amazon.com. Often you can play segments from the CD on your computer to hear sample music.

How do different sounds make you feel? Does jazz pick you up? Does classical music with a slow tempo make you sleepy, or does rock music give you anxiety or energize you? How do your body and mind react to the New Age or Alternative music? Some people have called blues "folk music for depressed people." When you are feeling "down," the prescription might be cheerful music or just the opposite, blues music to help you get in touch with your sad feelings and perhaps feel less alone, knowing that other people have problems and similar sadness.

Music artist Steven Halpern believes that most music (even classical) has been written to entertain rather than relax you. To find relaxing music look for music around 60 beats per minute. This will slow you and your heart down. (By Steve Halpern. "Why Musically Induced Alpha

Brainwaves are Good For You," ©1997, found at www.stevenhalpern.com.) Try out different music types and artists and look for what nourishes you.

Sight

You are nourished through your sense of sight. What was your favorite color in school? Everyone seems to have had one. Your favorite color was probably the crayon you used most. What colors do you like in your room? How do different colors make you feel in your gut? These answers are a key to what nourishes and soothes you.

Light is very important to many people's world. You may have heard about Seasonal Affective Disorder. SAD is a type of depression that can literally immobilize people who are the most sensitive to the decrease in light that occurs as the days shorten in winter. If you have mood changes that occur with season changes, check with your doctor. You may be able to get some help from an antidepressant, but there

> *The eyes are the window of the soul.*
>
> – Proverb

is much research that says full-spectrum lighting (which is different from fluorescent lighting) can greatly aid in diminishing the effects of reduced sunlight exposure in the winter. Full-spectrum lighting is available in the form of light boxes and as standard light bulbs. The book *Winter Blues: Seasonal Affective Disorder: What It Is and How To Overcome It* (New York: Guilford Press, 1998) is an excellent resource on the benefits of light therapy and SAD issues.

There are other areas where you can enhance what you see.

- Do you have a window near your favorite easy chair?

- Are you able to take a walk to view nature?

- Is your house decorated with colors that please you?

- Does clutter annoy you and are you able to remove such clutter from your sight?

These considerations are important if you spend a lot of time in a small place. Making your house cozy or bringing items from home to make your workspace more cheery can greatly enhance your mood.

Research has shown that patients whose hospital rooms have a view require less medication, are more content, and are able to leave the hospital sooner. Improving your view in the hospital may even make your managed care company happier! Maybe you cannot have the penthouse view at your hospital or at home, but you can still improve the space. We have rarely if ever had a hospital room with a view, but we have decorated our walls with cards. Carol remembers one hospital room she had in 1979 that looked out onto the roof of another part of the hospital. We do not think that area is used for rooms anymore, possibly because of the more recent research. Doug was in the hospital once on Thanksgiving Day. Our family tradition was to put up our Christmas tree on Thanksgiving weekend. Instead of putting up the family Christmas tree, Carol and Eric brought a Norfolk pine plant to Doug's hospital room. Although it wasn't quite the real thing, it lessened the sad feelings of helplessness we all were having that weekend.

Another vision enhancement is an aquarium. Perhaps you have seen one of these in your doctor's office. Your doctor may have one because research has shown that people who watch fish in an aquarium are able to reduce their blood pressure. Apparently a state of relaxation is induced from watching fish swim around in a tank. This state carries with it all of the health benefits of relaxation discussed earlier in Chapter Six, "Understanding Your Mind-Body Connection." If you don't have an aquarium, try focusing at a fire in the fireplace, watching the trees moving with the breeze outside your window, or watching the snow as each unique flake falls to the ground. All of these sights can induce a healthier state of mind and a happier, more content you, even just for awhile.

An oriental tradition, feng shui, is an interesting area to explore in regards to sight. According to feng shui consultant Paul Miller, feng shui has been used for over 3,000 years to order space in such ways that spirit or "chi" moves freely. Miller says that feng shui creates balanced, peaceful dwelling spaces where occupants can develop health and happiness. Rooms arranged according to feng shui feel open, safe, and balanced.

When we did some redecorating and furniture rearranging, we consulted with Miller. After making the changes that he suggested for our home, we had an immediate "ahhhhhh" feeling. The space felt more comfortable, more livable. Some might say, "easy." Although we have not explored the science behind feng shui, it worked for us and we enjoy our living area much more than before we made the changes. Paul Miller suggests several resources that can get you started with feng shui:

- *Feng Shui Made Easy: Designing Your Life with the Ancient Art of Placement*, by William Spear, New York: Harper, 1995.

- *Healing Environments: Your Guide to Indoor Well-Being*, by Carol Venolia, Berkeley, CA: Celestial Arts, 1988.

- *The Western Guide to Feng Shui,* by Kathryn Terah Collins, Ballantine Books, 1995.

Smell

Aromas have been used to promote healing by pleasing the sense of smell for many centuries. Examples include incense, perfume oils, and other scents which have been used for centuries to induce improved health and mood.

Various fragrances cause different reactions within us. Those who know how to mix them and use them can evoke relaxation, alertness, energy, romance, and sleep. Test out various scents for yourself. Is there one that reminds you of a time in childhood that makes you feel particularly safe? Does vanilla or cinnamon remind you of baking at home when you were young? Perhaps a certain perfume reminds you of early dates with your spouse or former lover. Fragrance oils may be used in the following ways including massage oil, perfume, diffuser mist, bath oil, or candles. There are certain oils that would not be appropriate to use under certain circumstances including high blood pressure, or pregnancy. We recommend two resources to start your learning about aromatherapy.

- *The Healing Aromatheraphy Bath*, by Margo Valentine Lazzara, C.Ht., Pownal, VT: Storey Books, 1999.

- *Aromatherapy Massage*, Clare Maxwell-Hudson, New York: DK Publishing, 1994.

Touch

Human beings cannot survive without touch. Early in this century, studies showed that a young child who was not touched and cuddled would die. Ornstein and Sobel tell the story of a physician named Fritz Talbot who visited the Children's Clinic in Dusseldorf, Germany in the 1940s. Dr. Talbot found the wards were clean, but something odd caught his attention. A large, elderly woman was lovingly carrying a sick baby on her hip. When questioned as to who she was, the medical director said, "Oh, that is Old Anna. When we have done everything we can medically for a baby, and it is still not doing well we turn it over to Old Anna, and she is always successful." (Robert Ornstein, Ph.D., and David Sobel, M.D., *Healthy Pleasures,* New York: Addison Wesley, 1989, p. 42.)

What an outstanding discovery! This finding led to new policies in caring for children in institutions, but as many of you know or remember, it took much longer for this to be instituted in hospital settings for many children and adults. Today, mothers of newborns have their babies with them from the moment they give birth. Sick children in a hospital are allowed to have a parent with them at all times and bed space is even available for both the parent and the child.

For adults, hospital back rubs and adult companions invited to stay with the patient are rare. Pressures to reduce cost have squeezed out the old-fashioned back rub even though it is widely believed that touch brings out the endorphins that can relieve pain. Fortunately, massage is becoming a way to relieve pain, at least temporarily, and to benefit people with certain muscular problems. Doug has found therapeutic massage to be one of the most effective ways to help manage his neck and shoulder pain. A few future-oriented medical plans are now including alternative approaches including therapeutic massage.

Knowing Your Talents and Gifts

One component of knowing yourself is recognizing what special strengths and talents you have. Whether you know it or not, you have characteristics that make you unique and special. They color how you will look at yourself and how you will accomplish what you want to do. These unique gifts are a key part of who you are.

We believe that each person is separately created and given special gifts and talents to be used in this world. No one can or should tell you who you are. Nobody except you can look inside you and decide what talents, traits, and passions you have. Everyone is unique. Being aware that you are uniquely you, with special gifts, talents, and passions may make life look brighter when all you see is what you have lost of yourself through life-changing illness.

Knowing and accepting yourself and your talents, traits, and passions can give you something positive on which to focus. When you use these talents, you will feel connected to a deep part within yourself because you are being true to your own self. Doing what you do well feels good.

There is a variety of ways to look at and categorize your talents, gifts and personality style. One way you can understand yourself better is realizing that you have multiple areas

> *I think that I shall never see*
> *A poem as lovely as a tree.*
>
> – Alfred Joyce Kilmer

of intelligence. Looking at intelligence as Harvard psychologist Howard Gardner does will rearrange how you think about the word "smart." Based on his pioneering research and theory in the area of multiple intelligences, Gardner's *Intelligence Reframed: Multiple Intelligences for the 21st Century* (New York: Basic Books, 1999) discusses nine intelligences that people have. These are distinct ways of being smart.

The modern Western culture we live in focuses most of its attention on highly articulate or logical areas of intelligence and tests primarily focus in these areas. Our culture tends to label people as smart or not so smart based almost entirely on how we can use words and numbers.

That's too bad. Even worse, we often use only this framework to look at ourselves.

Gardner has reframed and broadened how we look at the intelligence quotient (IQ) test which is commonly given to children in school. He recommends that you look at all of your capabilities and apply them in your everyday life. According to Gardner, being smart is not just a score on an IQ test. Rather it is your unique equation of the multiple intelligences mentioned above.

In his book *Seven Kinds of Smart: Identifying and Developing Your Many Intelligences*, Thomas Armstrong, Ph.D., describes these categories as word, logic and numbers, spatial, music, body-kinesthetic, interpersonal, and intrapersonal intelligences. (Plume: New York, 1999.) See figure of definitions on the following page for a more detailed description of these areas of multiple intelligences. (Please note that originally Dr. Armstrong and Dr. Gardner used seven intelligences in their research. They now believe that there are nine separate intelligences. The two new ones are nature and spiritual.)

Definitions of Multiple Intelligences

The following is a list from Gardner and Armstrong's research. The talents and virtues that comprise multiple intelligences and play a part in making you a unique person are described below.

Word. Involves sensitivity to spoken and written language, the ability to learn languages, and the capacity to use language in order to accomplish certain goals. This group includes lawyers, speakers, writers, and poets.

Logic and Numbers. Involves the capacity to analyze problems logically, carry out mathematical operations, and investigate issues scientifically. In this group you will find mathematicians, computer programmers, accountants, and scientists.

Spatial. Features the potential to recognize and manipulate the patterns of wide space as well as the patterns of more confined areas. This would include navigators, pilots, sculptors, surgeons, chess players, graphic artists and architects.

Music. This entails skill in performance, composition, and appreciation of musical patterns. Musicians of many kinds display this area of intelligence.

Body-Kinesthetic. Entails the potential of using one's whole body or parts of the body (like the hand) to solve problems or fashion products. This area includes people who are dancers, actors, athletes, craftspersons, and mechanics.

Interpersonal. This denotes a person's capacity to understand the intentions, motivations and desires of other people and consequently, to work effectively with others. People who need these skills include sales people, teachers, religious leaders, politicians, and actors.

Intrapersonal. This involves the capacity to understand oneself, to have an effective working model of oneself—including one's own desires, fears, and capacities—and to use such information effectively in regulating one's own life.

Nature. This person has expertise in the recognition and classification of the numerous species – the flora and fauna – of his or her environment. These are people who understand the living world.

Spiritual. Concern with ultimate life issues with respect to significant life questions such as meaning of life and of death.

You may wish to try this brief exercise. Number these intelligences from one to nine in the order you think applies to you. Notice both what your strongest and weakest areas are. Do you feel like you realized for the first time that you were smart? Many people do not realize that they are smart mostly because the world has not seen their areas of talents as intelligence.

As those of us with life-changing illness realize our strengths, we can find ways to exercise them and nurture ourselves. When Carol was first ill, she did a lot of hand needlework and became interested in photography. In exercising her intelligence and talents she received a sense of emotional calm and some immediate feedback about her self-worth.

Carol has a friend whose child has Down syndrome. His word and logic intelligences probably do not test very high on IQ tests compared to the general public. However, he is very happy and agreeable almost all of the time. His interpersonal intelligence is perhaps one of his higher intelligences. People with autism often have one area of intelligence that is extremely strong with little intelligence in most other areas. If you remember the movie *Rainman*, Raymond could solve complicated computations but was virtually unable to interact with other people.

Your life-changing illness may have changed what you are able to do. You may find it more difficult to do something that was once a strong area of intelligence. If you were very athletic and are now confined to a wheelchair, you no doubt find this confinement is a tremendous loss, and very frustrating. Losing some or all of your athletic abilities is naturally going to bring out strong feelings, including anger and grief. But when you are able to regain some perspective you may see a different way to use that intelligence. Consider the example of a "disabled" person who plays wheelchair basketball; this person has learned a different way to use his physical intelligence.

Christopher Reeve was once very active in many sports. Due to his paralysis, Reeve can no longer be physically active as he once was. He has used his fame and the admiration of his courage by others to create a well-organized and influential organization to raise money for research to find a cure for spinal cord injuries. Reeve is able to do this because of his strong social intelligence and ability to interact with people. He has formed many connections with people he knows in the entertainment business. He could have put his emotions into self-pity because he can no longer be physically active. This is not to say that he does not get discouraged because of his losses. Rather, he uses energy he might put to those negative emotions into something new and different that he can do well.

There are ways to exercise your growth areas. Is music low on your list? Take a music appreciation class at a community center. Do you have a picture deficit? Take an art or painting class. Don't worry if you are not perfect, you will not be graded. Try to feel good that you tried something that was a stretch for you. Remember that you have some stronger specialties. Everyone has his or her own strengths. By knowing and using your strengths, you can feel good about yourself, even if your area of intelligence was not measured in school.

Nobody except you can decide what is most important in your life. Everyone's gifts and passions are different and unique, but being aware that you "are uniquely you," with special gifts, talents, and passions will make life look brighter. This awareness can give you something inspiring to focus on when life-changing illness turns your life upside down.

Reaching Out to Others to Nurture Yourself

More than 100 years ago, Henry David Thoreau said, "It is one of the most beautiful compensations of this life that no man can sincerely try to help another without helping himself."

More recently, reaching out and helping someone has been proven to be beneficial to your health. In *The Healing Power of Doing Good*, author Allan Luks says he first noticed the benefits of "doing good" when he felt better after doing service projects and political activism when he was a young man. No doubt you have noticed how good you feel after doing something for someone else. It just feels good to help someone else.

Luks says, "It is the process of helping, without regard to its outcome, that is the healing factor. Regular helping of others can diminish the effects of disabling chronic pain and lessen the symptoms of physical distress." Luks' national survey resulted in the following observations which may help you see why he has come to the conclusion that helping others helps healing.

- The healthy helping syndrome has different phases.

- The "high" has clear and definite components.

- Phase two of the healthy helping syndrome brings a sense of calmness.

- People who experience the healthy helping syndrome have better perceived health.

- The health benefit returns whenever the helping act is remembered.

- The greater the frequency of volunteering, the greater the health benefits.

- Personal contact with the people being helped is important.

- Helper's high results most from helping people we don't know.

- Certain experiences are particularly effective (including community and societal projects).

- Men and women have an equal opportunity to benefit from this high.

(Allan Luks, with Peggy Payne, *The Healing Power of Doing Good,* Ballentine: New York, 1991, pp. 17-18.)

Although some people with life-changing illness may not be able to have personal contact if they are housebound due to symptoms caused by illness, almost everyone can find some way to reach out to another. Carol found that sending cards to people who were ill and writing them encouraging messages helped her to feel like she was doing something worthwhile even though she seldom left home and mostly saw people that were helping her. At another point in time she volunteered for a hotline which helped parents at risk for abusing their children. She was able to answer this phone line from her home. A friend of ours who has had several strokes and cannot drive gets a ride to church so she can help put the Sunday bulletin together.

You have your own unique restrictions on what you are able to do and what area of helping moves you to action. Finding a way to help others with similar problems can create a pronounced feeling of bonding between you and the other person. You may feel their pain more directly because you have already felt similar pain. The person being helped also feels this and knows that your help is based on a sincere interest in them. No matter what you choose to do, finding a creative way to help others is clearly beneficial both to the person you help and to you.

It is a fact that many people overdo themselves helping others. They sometimes become overburdened by helping. These people tend to be driven to achievement and perfection. They often have a need to please others and may have low self-esteem. Luks lists the following important factors for doing healthy helping. These factors are caution lights that everyone should use all the time, but especially when helping others.

- **Pace yourself.** The idea is to help others; but if you don't pace yourself, you may not be able to continue what you are doing.

- **Get help.** Get plenty of support, encouragement, and company for yourself. Teamwork is a way to learn from others and keep you from doing too much.

- **Start small.** Remember it is not necessary to rescue the whole world. In fact, do not kid yourself that you have the total responsibility for even one other person.

- **Do what is comfortable.** Explore what kind of helping is comfortable for you to do.

- **Do what you can.** Go ahead and do what you can (within the boundaries of your illness).

- **Quit if you have to.** Feel free to give up on a particular effort when you get into a situation that is not right for you.

- **Try again.** Do not quit helping because of one rejection, disappointment, or bad experience.

(Luks, pp. 150-154.)

By reaching out to other people you can find yourself feeling a little bit better. By implementing Luks' steps for self-care listed previously, you can help both yourself and someone else. The following is a list of ideas for how to help even if you have serious limitations.

- Send greeting cards to family or friends.

- Call a person who you know is lonely.

- Make creative gifts for others.

- Help at your place of worship.

- Volunteer for a nonprofit organization, possibly one that helps others with the same disease as yours.

This list is only a beginning. Do what excites you. Choose something within your ability but also do not be afraid to stretch and try something new to you. We are both amazed at what we are able to do when we reach outside of ourselves and help another.

Connecting with Others and Communicating Your Special Needs

Learning to accept compassion and assistance is far from automatic for most people. Yet people have a fundamental need and responsibility to help others. This can be hard to remember when you need to be on the asking end of helping. It is an important point to remember when people offer to help you with shopping, housecleaning, child care, or other ways that people who care about you want to provide you practical help and support. Nonetheless, as you can see from the above discussion on volunteering, when you ask for and receive help you are also helping someone else! Although it is possible to abuse other people's generosity, generally asking/giving help is a win-win experience for everyone.

In many of his books, including *Seven Habits of Effective Leaders*, author Dr. Stephen Covey describes the concept of interdependence as the most advanced and mature of relationships between people. You can be dependent (like an infant), independent (like a young adult) or interdependent, where you routinely ask for help and freely give help to others. When you have a life-changing illness, being interdependent can feel like lopsided dependence.

Asking and explaining to others what you need can actually give you choices that you would not otherwise have had. When someone asks to help you, remember that they need to be helping. Understanding other people's need to help can help you swallow useless pride and allow you to feel more comfortable asking for help. We have found that most people, including ourselves, want to help another person in need. However, knowing what people really need can be another story. If someone asks you if they can help you, give them some choices about what they might do to help you. That way, they know they are doing things that are truly helpful to you.

A minister once consoled Carol with a very deep but simple thought. He said, "Remember that people need to help each other. It is important for them to be able to help you. Take time to think about what you need and let them know when they ask." Following this hospital visit, someone from our church couple's group called to say our couples group wanted to help us with our household needs and chores. Carol remembers saying, "But I am not going to be getting better." The caller said that they would help as long as they were needed, and they did just that. Every time I went to the hospital, a couple of ladies would come and do a thorough cleaning of my house, someone else got our groceries every Saturday when they went shopping. Other people included Eric in their activities. Remember, just as helping another will help you, being helped can give you a feeling of empathy and support from others. Don't be ashamed to ask someone for help. Usually the person volunteering to help will do everything he or she can to be sure your needs are met.

Summary

You are unique and special, even in the midst of your life-changing illness. Taking good care of yourself is not selfish. You have not only the ability but the responsibility to take good care of yourself without feeling guilty about doing so. One of the hardest things to accept about taking care of yourself is that more often than not you should accept help that is offered by other people. You need to recognize that you benefit from their help, as does your family, and usually, the helper.

Nurturing yourself is a healthy prescription free of side effects, but it takes some effort. As we have described, consciously managing the time pie of your life, tapping into the power of your senses, knowing your talents and gifts, and reaching out to connect with others, are all part of the process. It may sound like a lot of work, but you're worth it!

If there is light in the soul,
There will be beauty in the person.
If there is beauty in the person,
There will be harmony in the house.
If there is harmony in the house,
There will be order in the nation.
If there is order in the nation,
There will be peace in the world.

– Chinese Proverb

Writing Your Next Chapter

The ideal day never comes. Today is ideal
for him who makes it so.

– Horatio W. Dresser

Now that you have read the first ten chapters, you know all about our stories, our philosophy, and the tools and resources that we have found useful to us and that we expect you to find helpful as well.

The next chapter is up to you. You have read how we came face to face with chronic illness more than 20 years ago, reaching the point where two roads diverged for us. We took the road that led us to find opportunities hidden within the crisis; friends, family and faith that we would not have otherwise discovered and inner strength and capabilities we would not have imagined having. That road eventually led us to write this book. We hope that road leads you to make a similar choice in your life to try to find the opportunity (Writing a book is optional!)

In the first part of the book, we dealt with navigating through the healthcare world, understanding your situation, building a partnership with your health care team, coping with hospitals, tests and medications and with the financial side of health care. We gave you our definition of life-changing illness:

The life of every man is a diary in which he means to write one story, and writes another.

– James Matthew Barrie

Life-changing illness is the result of diseases and/or conditions that are not necessarily life-threatening but have a dramatic, long-term impact on how you live your life.

We told you that we believe very strongly in the power of knowledge and self-care. Patients must play a key role in helping to shape and direct their medical treatment. We know from our own experience how easy it is to become passive and to be "taken care of" when we are very sick. We even offered you a new definition for patient:

> pa tient (pa' shent) n. 1 a well-informed person who seeks knowledge, forms an effective partnership with doctors and other healthcare professionals and makes decisions which help to shape his or her treatment.

We offered suggestions and shared feelings and experiences we have had as patients working with doctors and other healthcare professionals and as hospital patients.

The second half of the book is a resource for learning how to integrate the various dimensions of your life with life-changing illness, helping you to become a whole person. We started with key components of taking care of your body, many of which apply whether or not you deal with illness. We shared with you our firm belief in the mysterious and powerful links between the mind, body, and spirit in the healing process. We explored ways to help you find your purpose, realign your attitude, and nurture yourself and take care of your biological you. We described in detail specific ways to nurture each of these dimensions.

> *The strongest principle of growth lies in human choice.*
>
> – George Eliot

We acknowledged up front that we do not have all the answers and that we do not know you personally. Only one person really knows you. You. So you must be the author of your next chapter. We hope that you find this book to be a helpful resource for you and that it helps you live at least a little better, even if you can't get well. We would love to hear your stories and get your feedback. Send your stories to Patient Corner at our Web site, www.patientpress.com, where you will find books, other publications, and links to other resources. We wish you well.

About the Authors

Carol J. Langenfeld, M.S.Ed., L.P.C.

Carol Langenfeld, co-author of *Living Better: Every Patient's Guide for Living with Illness,* is a Licensed Professional Counselor with an M.S.Ed. in Counseling from the University of Dayton in 1996. Carol completed the Clinical Training in Mind/Body Medicine program at Harvard Medical School's Mind/Body Medical Institute in 1999. She also completed the National Institute of Clinical Behavioral Medicine's Advanced Training Certification Program in Mind/Body Medicine in 1995. Carol is a National Certified Counselor and is a member of the American Counseling Association.

Carol has lived with sclerderma, a serious connective tissue disease, since 1979, when she was the young mother of an 18-month old son. Her illness has resulted in many medical crises and close calls, including cardiac arrests and serious arrhythmias.

Douglas E. Langenfeld, M.B.A., C.P.A., F.H.F.M.A.

Doug Langenfeld is a Certified Public Accountant who retired for health reasons from Ernst & Young, an international consulting firm, where he was a partner serving healthcare clients for more than 20 years. Doug earned an M.B.A. in Finance from Miami University, Oxford, Ohio, in 1975. He is also a Fellow, Healthcare Financial Management Association. Doug has a part-time investment and financial planning practice. He enjoys writing and has received regional awards for several of his essays.

In addition to being Carol's husband, Doug has lived with his own serious illness since discovery of a pituitary tumor in 1991. The tumor required surgery, radiation treatments, and long-term medications. His condition, called acromegaly, has resulted in continuing endocrine system complications.

More About the Authors

Carol and Doug Langenfeld came face-to-face with illness in 1979. With "a lot of help from their friends," they made a choice to find opportunity hidden within the crisis of Carol's illness. Carol says, "We found friends, family, and faith that we may not have discovered. We found inner strength and capabilities we could not have imagined. We certainly never expected to write a book!"

Carol and Doug view theirs and others' chronic illnesses as "life-changing." They believe in the power of knowledge and self-care and that patients need to participate actively in shaping their life changes. The authors' experience as patients has led them to see the importance of patients being informed, active participants in their health care. They also firmly believe in the mysterious and powerful links between the mind, body, and spirituality as a key part of the healing process. They plan to write a series of books and find other ways to be a source for information to inform, nurture, and empower other patients. Look for Carol's next books, *Giving Your Attitude Wings: Every Patient's Guide to Developing a Healthy Attitude*, and *Living Better with Scleroderma: Every Patient's Guide*, and Doug's next book, *Career, Interrupted: Reconnecting When Illness Short Circuits Your Career*, in the near future.

INDEX

PATIENT PRESS

6475 Perimeter Drive, Box 110
Dublin, Ohio 43016
Phone 614/799-1444 • Fax 614/799-1448
www.patientpress.com • langenfeld@patientpress.com
SAN: 253-3685

Providing information to equip people living with
illness to be informed and empowered to be in control
of their health care and their lives.

You can live better even if your body can't get well!

Order Form

E-mail orders: orders@patientpress.com.
Fax orders: 614/799-1448. Send this form
Telephone orders: Call 614/799-1444 or toll-free order line (1-866/799-1444). Have your credit card number ready.
Postal orders: Patient Press, 6475 Perimeter Drive, Box 110, Dublin, OH 43016. USA.

Please send the following:
_____ copies of <u>Living Better: Every Patient's Guide to Living with Illness</u> at $14.95 per copy.

Name:_____

Address:_____

_____

City:_____

State:_____Zip:_____

Telephone:_____

E-mail address:_____

Sales tax: Please add 5.75% for items shipped to Ohio addresses.

Shipping: Please add $4.50 for the first item and $2.00 for each additional item shipped to the USA. For items shipped outside the USA, please add $9.00 for the first item and $5.00 for each additional item.

Total order:
# of copies _____ times $14.95 per copy   _____
Ohio sales tax   5.75% if shipped to Ohio   _____
Shipping   See above instructions   _____
TOTAL   _____

Payment: [ ]Check, [ ]MasterCard, [ ]Visa, [ ]American Express
Card number:_____
Name on card:_____
Expiration date:_____/_____

Visit www.patientpress.com

PATIENT PRESS

6475 Perimeter Drive, Box 110
Dublin, Ohio 43016
Phone 614/799-1444 • Fax 614/799-1448
www.patientpress.com • langenfeld@patientpress.com
SAN: 253-3685

Providing information to equip people living with
illness to be informed and empowered to be in control
of their health care and their lives.

You can live better even if your body can't get well!

Order Form

E-mail orders: orders@patientpress.com.

Fax orders: 614/799-1448. Send this form

Telephone orders: Call 614/799-1444 or toll-free order line (1-866/799-1444). Have your credit card number ready.

Postal orders: Patient Press, 6475 Perimeter Drive, Box 110, Dublin, OH 43016. USA.

Please send the following:

_____ copies of <u>Living Better: Every Patient's Guide to Living with Illness</u> at $14.95 per copy.

Name:_____

Address:_____

_____

City:_____

State:_____Zip:_____

Telephone:_____

E-mail address:_____

Sales tax: Please add 5.75% for items shipped to Ohio addresses.

Shipping: Please add $4.50 for the first item and $2.00 for each additional item shipped to the USA. For items shipped outside the USA, please add $9.00 for the first item and $5.00 for each additional item.

Total order:

# of copies _____	times $14.95 per copy	_____
Ohio sales tax	5.75% if shipped to Ohio	_____
Shipping	See above instructions	_____
TOTAL		_____

Payment: [ ]Check, [ ]MasterCard, [ ]Visa, [ ]American Express

Card number:_____

Name on card:_____

Expiration date:_____/_____

Visit www.patientpress.com